T0383248

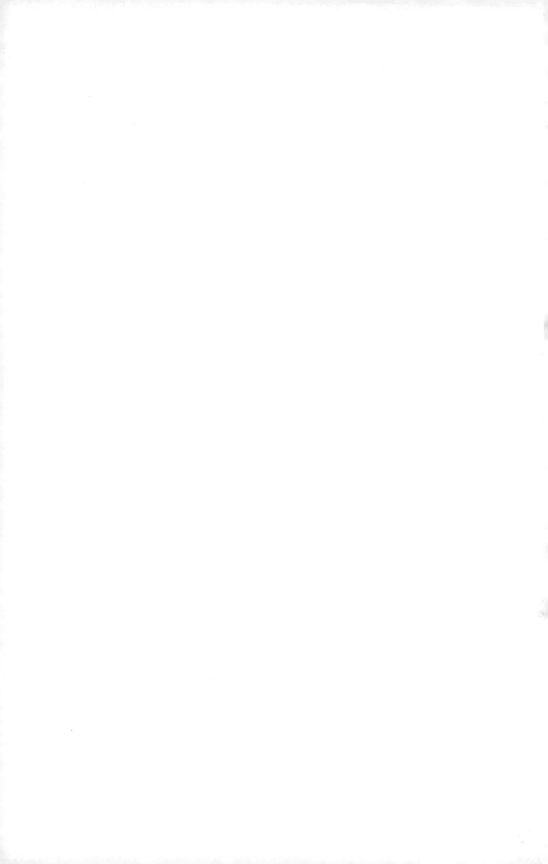

Pediatrics

Editor

PATRICIA V. BURKHART

NURSING CLINICS
OF NORTH AMERICA

www.nursing.theclinics.com

Consulting Editor
STEPHEN D. KRAU

June 2013 • Volume 48 • Number 2

ELSEVIER

1600 John F. Kennedy Boulevard • Suite 1800 • Philadelphia, Pennsylvania, 19103-2899

http://www.theclinics.com

NURSING CLINICS OF NORTH AMERICA Volume 48, Number 2
June 2013 ISSN 0029-6465, ISBN-13: 978-1-4557-7126-4

Editor: Katie Saunders
Developmental Editor: Donald Mumford

Nursing Clinics of North America (ISSN 0029-6465) is published quarterly by Elsevier Inc., 360 Park Avenue South, New York, NY 10010-1710. Months of issue are March, June, September, and December. Periodicals postage paid at New York, NY and additional mailing offices. Subscription price per year is, $144.00 (US individuals), $374.00 (US institutions), $260.00 (international individuals), $456.00 (international institutions), $210.00 (Canadian individuals), $456.00 (Canadian institutions), $79.00 (US students), and $129.00 (international students). To receive student/resident rate, orders must be accompanied by name of affiliated institution, date of term, and the signature of program/residency coordinator on institution letterhead. Orders will be billed at individual rate until proof of status is received. Foreign air speed delivery is included in all *Clinics* subscription prices. All prices are subject to change without notice. **POSTMASTER:** Send address changes to *Nursing Clinics*, Elsevier Health Sciences Division, Subscription Customer Service, 3251 Riverport Lane, Maryland Heights, MO 63043. **Customer Service: Telephone: 1-800-654-2452** (U.S. and Canada); **1-314-447-8871 (outside U.S. and Canada). Fax: 1-314-447-8029.** E-mail: journalscustomerservice-usa@elsevier.com (for print support) and **journalsonlinesupport-usa@elsevier.com** (for online support).

Nursing Clinics of North America is covered in *EMBASE/Excerpta Medica, MEDLINE/PubMed (Index Medicus), Social Sciences Citation Index, Current Contents, ASCA, Cumulative Index to Nursing, RNdex Top 100,* and Allied Health Literature and International Nursing Index (INI).

Printed and bound by CPI Group (UK) Ltd, Croydon, CR0 4YY
Transferred to Digital Printing, 2013

Contributors

CONSULTING EDITOR

STEPHEN D. KRAU, PhD, RN, CNE
Associate Professor, Vanderbilt University School of Nursing, South Nashville, Tennessee

EDITOR

PATRICIA V. BURKHART, PhD, RN
Professor and Associate Dean for Undergraduate Studies, University of Kentucky, Lexington, Kentucky

AUTHORS

SARAH ADKINS, MSC
College of Justice and Safety, Eastern Kentucky University, Richmond, Kentucky

MOLLIE E. ALESHIRE, DNP, FNP-BC, PNP-BC
Assistant Professor, College of Nursing, University of Kentucky, Lexington, Kentucky

H. JORGE BALUARTE, MD
Division of Nephrology, The Children's Hospital of Philadelphia, Perelman School of Medicine, University of Pennsylvania, Philadelphia, Pennsylvania

BARBARA L. BEACHAM, MSN, RN
Doctoral Candidate, Center for Health Equity Research, University of Pennsylvania School of Nursing, Philadelphia, Pennsylvania

MELISSA H. BELLIN, PhD, LCSW
Associate Professor, School of Social Work, The University of Maryland at Baltimore, Baltimore, Maryland

PATRICIA V. BURKHART, PhD, RN
Professor and Associate Dean for Undergraduate Studies, University of Kentucky, Lexington, Kentucky

ARLENE M. BUTZ, ScD, MSN
Professor, Department of Pediatrics, The Johns Hopkins University School of Medicine; School of Nursing, Baltimore, Maryland

JANET A. DEATRICK, PhD, FAAN
Professor and Co-Director, Center for Health Equity Research, University of Pennsylvania School of Nursing, Philadelphia, Pennsylvania

RITA DOUMIT, PhD, RN
Instructor, University of Lebanon Beirut Campus

ELIZABETH A. ELY, PhD, RN
Nurse Researcher, Department of Nursing, The Children's Hospital of Philadelphia, Philadelphia, Pennsylvania

RACHEL FARMER, MS, RN
Family Nurse Practitioner, Minute Clinic, Knoxville, Tennessee

KEVIN D. FRICK, PhD
Professor, Department of Health Policy and Management, The Johns Hopkins University Bloomberg School of Public Health, Baltimore, Maryland

CARRIE GORDY, APRN, MSN
Pediatric Nurse Practitioner, Assistant Professor, University of Kentucky College of Nursing; Pediatric Nurse Practitioner, Family Care Center Pediatric Clinic, Lexington, Kentucky

RENEE C. GREEN, BSN, RN
Staff Nurse, Department of Nursing, The Children's Hospital of Philadelphia, Philadelphia, Pennsylvania

PATRICK R. HARRISON, BS, MA
Department of Psychology, Loyola University Chicago, Chicago, Illinois

VICKI HENSLEY, MSN, APRN
College of Nursing, Lecturer, University of Kentucky, Lexington, Kentucky

BRENDA M. HOLTZER, PhD, RN
Pediatric Clinical Nurse Specialist-Board Certified, Assistant Professor and Coordinator of the RN-BS Program, Penn State Abington, Abington, Pennsylvania

YU HUANG, MS
Doctoral Student, Department of Industrial and Systems Engineering, College of Engineering, University of Tennessee, Knoxville, Tennessee

LYNNE A. JENSEN, PhD, APRN
Associate Professor, College of Nursing, University of Kentucky, Lexington, Kentucky

SARA L. JONES, PhD, RN
Clinical Assistant Professor, College of Nursing, University of Arkansas for Medical Sciences, Little Rock, Arkansas

JOANNE KOUBA
Assistant Professor, Niehoff School of Nursing, Loyola University Chicago, Chicago, Illinois

JOAN KUB, PhD, MSN
Associate Professor, Department of Community Health, School of Nursing, Baltimore, Maryland

BRENDA KUNS, RN
Nurse Manager, Family Care Center, Pediatric Clinic, Lexington, Kentucky

XUEPING LI, PhD
Associate Professor, Director, Ideation Laboratory, Department of Industrial and Systems Engineering, College of Engineering, University of Tennessee; Co-Director, Health Information Technology and Simulation Lab, Department of Industrial and Systems Engineering, College of Engineering, University of Tennessee, Knoxville, Tennessee

MEI-LIN CHEN LIM, BSN, RN
Certified Clinical Research Coordinator, Senior Nurse Research Coordinator, Department of Nursing, The Children's Hospital of Philadelphia, Philadelphia, Pennsylvania

TERRI H. LIPMAN, PhD, CRNP, FAAN
Division of Endocrinology and Diabetes, The Children's Hospital of Philadelphia, University of Pennsylvania School of Nursing, Philadelphia, Pennsylvania

SHARON E. LOCK, PhD, APRN
Associate Professor, College of Nursing, University of Kentucky, Lexington, Kentucky

AMY MANION, PhD, RN, CPNP
Instructor, College of Nursing, Rush University, Chicago, Illinois

KRISTYN L. MICKLEY, BSN, RN
Undergraduate Baccalaureate Nursing Student, College of Nursing, University of Kentucky; Pediatric Intensive Care Nurse, Kentucky Children's Hospital, Lexington, Kentucky

LISA K. MILITELLO, MSN, MPH, CPNP
College of Nursing, Arizona State University, Phoenix, Arizona

KATHLEEN A. MONTGOMERY, MSN, CRNP
Division of Endocrinology and Diabetes, The Children's Hospital of Philadelphia, Philadelphia, Pennsylvania

KATHRYN M. MURPHY, PhD, RN
Division of Endocrinology and Diabetes, The Children's Hospital of Philadelphia, University of Pennsylvania School of Nursing, Philadelphia, Pennsylvania

SARAH J. RATCLIFFE, PhD
Department of Biostatistics and Epidemiology, Perelman School of Medicine, University of Pennsylvania, Philadelphia, Pennsylvania

MARY KAY RAYENS, PhD
Professor, College of Nursing and College of Public Health, University of Kentucky, Lexington, Kentucky

DELANNA REED, PhD
Instructor, Storytelling Program, East Tennessee State University, Johnson City, Tennessee

CHERYL K. SCHMIDT, PhD, RN, CNE
Academy of Nursing Education Fellow, Associate Professor, College of Nursing, University of Arkansas for Medical Sciences, Little Rock, Arkansas

LESLIE K. SCOTT, PhD, PNP-BC, CDE
Assistant Professor, College of Nursing, PNP Track Coordinator, University of Kentucky, Lexington, Kentucky

SUSAN T. SHAFFER, RN
Staff Nurse, Department of Nursing, The Children's Hospital of Philadelphia, Philadelphia, Pennsylvania

APRIL N. SIGLER, BA
PhD Student, School Psychology, College of Education, University of Kentucky, Lexington, Kentucky

ANNA OLAFIA SIGURDARDOTTIR, MSc, RN
PhD (Student), Clinical Nurse Specialist and Clinical Assistant Professor at Landspitali - The National University hospital in Iceland; University of Iceland, Reykjavik, Iceland

ERLA KOLBRUN SVAVARSDOTTIR, PhD, RN
Faculty of Nursing, Professor, School of Health Sciences, University of Iceland; Head of Research and Development of Family Nursing, Landspitali - The National University Hospital, Reykjavik, Iceland

BARBARA VELSOR-FRIEDRICH, PhD, RN
Professor and Faculty Scholar, Niehoff School of Nursing, Loyola University Chicago, Chicago, Illinois

STEVEN WILLI, MD
Division of Endocrinology and Diabetes, The Children's Hospital of Philadelphia, Perelman School of Medicine, University of Pennsylvania, Philadelphia, Pennsylvania

TAMI H. WYATT, PhD, RN
Associate Professor, Chair, Educational Technology and Simulation, Co-Director, Health Information Technology and Simulation Lab, College of Nursing, University of Tennessee, Knoxville, Tennessee

COLLEEN D. ZARNOWSKY, BSN, RN
Staff Nurse, Department of Nursing, The Children's Hospital of Philadelphia, Philadelphia, Pennsylvania

Contents

support increased significantly for mothers in the experimental group. The children of the parents in the experimental group reported significantly lower problems with asthma treatment on the treatment problems sub-scale of the asthma QOL scale after the intervention. These results highlight the benefit of therapeutic conversations for families of children and adolescent with asthma to support or enhance QOL.

Health care autonomy typically occurs during late adolescence but health care providers and families often expect children with chronic health conditions to master self-care earlier. Few studies have examined the development of health care autonomy as it pertains to self-care and family management. This review links the 3 concepts and discusses the implications for families and health care providers. Case studies are provided as exemplars to highlight areas where intervention and research is needed.

Chronic conditions can affect school-age children in more ways than just physically. Normal childhood maturation is critical at this age, yet daily management of chronic symptoms can be challenging. This article describes 4 common childhood chronic illnesses (asthma, seizure disorders, diabetes, and cystic fibrosis), and the impact these conditions have on the developing child. Self-efficacy, the belief that one can effectively perform necessary skills, is essential to self-management of chronic conditions and contributes in a positive way to the child's normal development. Implications for clinical practice and future research are discussed.

The goal of managing diabetes in childhood is to assist the child in becoming a physically healthy and emotionally mature adult, free from complications associated with diabetes. Gradual achievement of self-care independence occurs as developmental changes evolve during childhood. Inappropriate expectations related to self-care competence may lead to impaired diabetes control. It is important to have an understanding of child development and cognitive development in order ensure adequate expectations of self-care skill acquisition and the appropriate transition of self-care skills. Numerous steps can be taken to assist the child with diabetes in attaining developmentally appropriate, self-management skills.

Evidence-based practice is a shift in the health care culture from basing decisions on consensus opinion, past practice, and precedent toward the use of rigorous analysis of scientific evidence using outcomes research and clinical evidence to guide clinical decision making. The development of evidence-based clinical practice guidelines (CPG) is critical to guide the assessment and management of children with diabetes. This article provides an overview of the infrastructure and processes that are crucial to providing evidence-based care in a large urban pediatric diabetes center. Development of a CPG to identify microalbuminuria in children with type 1 diabetes is discussed.

Susan T. Shaffer, Colleen D. Zarnowsky, Renee C. Green, Mei-Lin Chen Lim, Brenda M. Holtzer, and Elizabeth A. Ely

This article presents the bedside nurses' perspectives on their experience with conducting an evidence based practice project. This is especially important in the climate of hospitals working to achieve Magnet Recognition. The facilitators and barriers to project design and completion are discussed in detail. Strategies to overcome barriers are presented. Facilitators for bedside nurses include motivation and professional development. Most common barriers were lack of time and limited knowledge about the process. Interventions aimed at research utilization can be successful when mindful of commonly understood barriers to project completion with steps taken to resolve those barriers.

NURSING CLINICS OF NORTH AMERICA

FORTHCOMING ISSUES

September 2013
Addictions
Al Rundio, PhD, DNP, RN,
APRN, NEA-BC, DPNAP, *Editor*

December 2013
Genomics
Stephen D. Krau, PhD, RN, CNE, *Editor*

RECENT ISSUES

March 2013
Asthma
Catherine D. Catrambone, PhD, RN, FAAN,
and Linda M. Follenweider, MS, APN,
C-FNP, *Editors*

December 2012
New Directions in Nursing Education
Mary Ellen Smith Glasgow, PhD, RN,
ACNS-BC, *Editor*

September 2012
Second Generation QSEN
Joanne Disch, PhD, RN, FAAN, and
Jane Barnsteiner, PhD, RN, FAAN, *Editors*

Preface

Current Challenges in Pediatrics

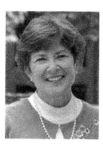

Patricia V. Burkhart, PhD, RN
Editor

We often hear the phrase "children are not miniature adults." This means that general nursing strategies and protocols developed for adults do not necessarily support positive health outcomes for children. There has been significant progress in our understanding of the pathophysiology and in the advancement of treatment modalities of current health challenges in pediatrics. However, education and nursing care must be tailored appropriately to the developmental level of the child and the readiness of the family to provide the caretaking needs at home.

This issue of *Nursing Clinics of North America* provides an overview of evidence-based nursing strategies for children of various ages and diagnoses. It covers an age group ranging from infancy to adolescence. The majority of the topics address chronic conditions and the long-term implications impacting children's normal development and mastery of age-related tasks. The pediatric challenges covered in this issue include pediatric abusive head trauma; adolescent sexually transmitted diseases; the impact of bullying and natural disasters on children; and coping with chronic diseases such as asthma and diabetes. Most of the articles incorporate developmental needs of specific age groups and include evidence-based nursing protocols to promote positive health outcomes for children and their families.

The specific health condition and age group create different types of challenges. In addition, the family must be considered part of the treatment plan, in varying degrees, depending on the age and specific needs of the child. Infants rely solely on their caregivers, trusting their needs will be met. Toddlers, developing a sense of autonomy, may regress in their normal tasks if treatment regimens require control of daily activities and limit setting. Preschool children, achieving a sense of initiative in mastering their world, still have little understanding of their illness but are aware of their bodies and want some control over daily management. School-aged children are becoming increasing independent, more communicative, and socially involved. When provided with necessary

Nurs Clin N Am 48 (2013) xiii–xiv
http://dx.doi.org/10.1016/j.cnur.2013.03.001
0029-6465/13/$ – see front matter © 2013 Published by Elsevier Inc.

skills, they are able to handle some of the care management themselves. Adolescence is a transitional time between childhood and adulthood. Adolescents want to be part of the decision-making and goal design. It is a time for them to assume most of the care management responsibility, with less parental support; however, adolescents need successful experiences managing their health to have positive outcomes.

Several of the authors in this issue (eg, Beacham and Deatrick; Mickley, Burkhart, and Sigler; and Scott) offer insights into gradually transitioning the responsibility and management of the condition-specific treatments to the child. There is a need for developmentally appropriate protocols to meet the physiologic and psychosocial needs of children and to provide opportunities for children to learn self-management skills. Often the research conducted provides little attention to theoretically based studies, particularly the utilization of developmental theory for managing childhood conditions and measuring children's health outcomes, including quality of life.

The authors contributing to this issue of *Nursing Clinics of North America* have dedicated their lives to the health and well-being of children, including children with long-term health conditions. These pediatric experts are developing cutting-edge, evidence-based protocols specifically for children and their families. While progress has been made in this area, more is needed to advance effective educational strategies and scientifically based interventions for assisting children and their families to successfully manage their health conditions. These protocols need to be developmentally and culturally sensitive for managing long-term conditions at home. I applaud our pediatric nursing champions for their dedication to this important work and for contributing their expertise in addressing current pediatric challenges central to this issue of *Nursing Clinics of North America.*

Patricia V. Burkhart, PhD, RN
202-D College of Nursing
University of Kentucky
751 Rose Street
Lexington, KY 40536-0232, USA

E-mail address:
patricia.burkhart@uky.edu

Pediatric Abusive Head Trauma

Carrie Gordy, APRN, MSN[a,b,*], Brenda Kuns, RN[b]

KEYWORDS

- Abusive head trauma • Shaken baby syndrome • Child maltreatment • Child abuse

KEY POINTS

- PAHT is a significant cause of morbidity and mortality in the United States.
- Many infants and young children die from PAHT injuries and others sustain life-altering neurologic damage.
- Healthcare providers need to increase their knowledge base and level of suspicion when confronted with common vague presenting symptoms, such as vomiting, irritability, and feeding difficulties.
- Early recognition and appropriate action may significantly improve outcomes for victims of PAHT.
- Any provider who has reason to suspect abuse has a legal and moral obligation to take the steps necessary to protect the child.
- Comprehensive community-based programs that teach caregivers the dangers of shaking and strategies for coping with infant crying may hold the best hope for reducing the incidence of PAHT.

INTRODUCTION

Child maltreatment may be reaching epidemic proportions. In the United States, a child abuse report is made every 10 seconds. Statistics indicate more than 3.3 million reports, involving approximately 6 million children, are made annually resulting in an estimated annual cost of $120 billion.[1] Furthermore, with more than five deaths daily, the United States leads all industrialized nations in pediatric abuse-related deaths.[2,3] Among all forms of physical child abuse, head trauma is the leading cause of death and disability.[4] Abuse is the third leading cause of head injury among children in the United States and is the leading cause of serious head injuries in the first year of life.[5] It is crucial that nurses be proficient in the recognition of children who are at risk for this type of abuse and that they be able to identify early signs and symptoms in those who have already been victimized. Pediatric abusive head trauma (PAHT) fatalities are believed by many experts to be 100% preventable through early

Disclosures: None.
[a] University of Kentucky College of Nursing, 315 CON Building, Rose Street, Lexington, KY 40504–0232, USA; [b] Family Care Center Pediatric Clinic, 1135 Red Mile Place, Lexington, KY 40504, USA
* Corresponding author.
E-mail address: Cgordy1@uky.edu

recognition of risk factors, early identification and prompt intervention, and educational preventative programs. Nurses play a critical role in the development and implementation of prevention programs.

WHAT IS PAHT?

Abusive head trauma refers to any intentionally inflicted injury to the head or neck, including cranial, cerebral, and spinal injuries. The mechanism of injury may be blunt force trauma, shaking, throwing, dropping, slamming, violent pulling, or any combination of these.[6,7] The term "shaken baby syndrome" is well recognized and commonly used to describe inflicted head trauma in small children. Recognizing the limitations of this term, specifically that all inflicted head trauma is not the result of shaking, the American Academy of Pediatrics currently recommends that the term "abusive head trauma" instead be used.[7] The term abusive head trauma includes shaken baby syndrome, shaken impact syndrome, and all other forms of inflicted head trauma.

EPIDEMIOLOGY

As with all forms of child maltreatment, the actual incidence of PAHT is difficult to quantify. Available statistics only partially represent the actual number of cases. This is caused in part by the criminal nature of the act and the failure of healthcare providers to recognize the syndrome and report it appropriately. Further complicating the issue has been the lack of uniform definitions and terminology. In April 2012, the Centers for Disease Control and Prevention addressed this problem by issuing recommended definitions for public health surveillance and research related to PAHT.[5]

Currently available information identifies PAHT as the leading cause of death from child abuse in the United States.[8] Between 1000 and 1500 known cases occur annually. Of these approximately 20% of victims sustain minor injuries, whereas 50% result in life-altering neurologic damage. Thirty percent of victims die as a result of their injuries.[9] PAHT accounts for 64% of all head injuries in infants younger than 12 months and 95% of the serious intracranial injuries in infants younger than 12 months. Approximately 10% of all child abuse deaths are from PAHT. The highest incidence occurs between the ages of 3 and 8 months of age. Although uncommon after the age of 2 years, cases have been reported up to 5 years of age.[10,11]

MECHANISMS OF INJURY

Pediatric nurses fully understand that "children are not small adults." This is particularly true when considering head trauma. Infants are especially vulnerable to the effects of head trauma for several reasons:

1. Relative to their bodies an infant's head is large, heavy, and unstable. By the age of 2 years, a child's brain has grown to 75% of its full adult size and weight.[8,12,13]
2. The musculature of the infant's neck is weak and underdeveloped making the head unstable and more susceptible to the movement associated with acceleration-deceleration forces.[8,12,13]
3. The infant's brain has a water content of 88% (compared with the 77% in adult brains). This coupled with incomplete myelination results in brain tissue that is softer and more vulnerable to acceleration-deceleration and shear injury.[8,12,13]
4. The thin, pliable infant skull and shallow subarachnoid space allows for more effective transfer of forces to the brain.[8,12,13]
5. Greater cerebral blood volume maximizes the potential for bleeding and swelling in the brain.[8,12,13]

The mechanism of injury is from direct blunt force trauma, shaking, throwing, dropping, slamming, violently pulling, or any combination of these. Most cases and those with the gravest outcomes are believed to be the result of violent shaking or violent shaking followed by slamming the infant onto a solid surface.[14] Forceful, vigorous shaking of an infant or young child results in the head rotating uncontrollably about the neck. This vigorous movement causes the brain to bounce against the skull rupturing blood vessels, tearing nerves, and bruising delicate brain tissue. The forceful squeezing of the child during the shaking episode impedes venous return and forces more blood into the brain. This raises intravascular pressure and increases the potential for vascular rupture and bleeding in the brain. The damage is further exacerbated by bleeding and swelling occurring after the initial injury further increasing the pressure on blood vessels and brain tissue. Damage can occur in a matter of seconds from as few as three violent shakes.[15–17]

RISK FACTORS

PAHT occurs across all socioeconomic levels and among all ethnic groups. The trigger for most episodes of abuse seems to be caregiver frustration related to an infant's prolonged, inconsolable crying.[11,12,18] Although it is impossible to identify every potential victim before the occurrence of abuse, healthcare providers who are knowledgeable about the risk factors may be able to improve intervention strategies and outcomes. Identifiable characteristics that place an infant or small child at increased risk include but are not limited to poor bonding, neonatal abstinence syndrome, colic, small birth weight or prematurity, chronic illness or disability, and difficult temperament.[11,12,18]

Statistics indicate that certain personal or family characteristics also increase abuse potential. Perpetrators of PAHT have long been believed to be primarily male. Recent studies, however, have called this assumption into question. One study looked at 34 cases of PAHT over a period of 10 years and found male and female perpetrators in equal proportions.[19] The investigators concluded that although females are just as likely as males to commit PAHT, the male perpetrators were usually younger, more likely to confess and be convicted, and were more likely to inflict serious harm on the victims.[19]

Other characteristics believed to make an adult more prone to abuse include a history of domestic violence, having been abused themselves as a child, being a single parent, social isolation and a lack of a support system, limited coping mechanisms, poor self-esteem, substance abuse, financial stress, and having unrealistic expectations of the child.[16,18,20] Several studies have linked the current economic downturn to an increase in child maltreatment,[21] making it more important than ever for all types of healthcare providers to be informed and alert for indicators of abuse.

INJURIES ASSOCIATED WITH PAHT

The types of injuries sustained from PAHT are many and varied. They range from minor injuries that go undetected to life-threatening injuries. In addition to the primary injury sustained directly from the traumatic forces, the brain is often secondarily damaged by ischemia and hypoxia.[22] In abused children the extent of cerebral injury may be more closely associated with the secondary ischemic-hypoxic injury than with the primary injury. Various mechanisms contributing to hypoxia include apnea from brainstem injury, spinal cord injury, prolonged seizure activity, or loss of airway.[23,24]

Cranial injuries associated with PAHT include closed head injury (concussion); subdural hematoma or hemorrhage; retinal hemorrhages; central nervous system or spinal cord injury; and death.[25] Associated injuries are not always present but may include skull or neck fractures, posterior rib fractures from gripping the chest during shaking, long bone fractures from searing injury, traumatic alopecia, and black eyes.[14,20,21] Consequences of these traumatic brain injuries include learning disabilities, vision impairment, total blindness, speech and hearing loss, cerebral palsy, persistent vegetative state, and death.[14,20,21]

PRESENTING SIGNS AND SYMPTOMS

Presenting signs and symptoms of PAHT are frequently vague and nonspecific, mimicking other common pediatric conditions. Depending on the severity, some cases may never be seen by a healthcare provider, whereas others present no symptoms until they enter school and the children are found to have behavioral problems or learning disabilities.[3,15,16,26] Parents may fail to disclose or may even be unaware of the traumatic incident making recognition of head trauma abuse challenging. Children with significant injury may present with apnea, often referred to as the cardinal sign; seizures; or coma.[25,27] Less severe injuries are more difficult to recognize because the presenting symptoms point to numerous other conditions. Such complaints as vomiting, fever, irritability, lethargy, poor suck or swallow, decreased smiling or vocalization, poor head control or a change in head control ability, increasing head circumference, and failure to focus or track may be early warning signs of increased intracranial pressure caused by head injury.[14,26] Studies show that healthcare providers are less likely to associate these symptoms with abuse in very young patients with both parents in the home.[26] It is important that all healthcare providers consider carefully the possibility of abusive head trauma when evaluating a young child with any one or a combination of these symptoms.

Although no intervention is likely to significantly alter the outcome with severe traumatic brain injury, early recognition and aggressive treatment may prevent the secondary progressive hypoxic ischemic damage in milder cases.[15] Moreover, identification of very mild injury and appropriate intervention may prevent the child from being more seriously injured in the future. A retrospective study of 173 cases of serious abusive head trauma in children younger than age 3 years suggested that 31.2% of the cases (N = 54) had been misdiagnosed by a physician between the abusive episode and the eventual diagnosis. The children in this study were evaluated between two and nine times between the time of initial injury and eventual diagnosis. According to their findings, the average time between injury and diagnosis was 1 week. The researchers concluded that four out of five deaths might have been prevented by earlier recognition.[26]

PREVENTION STRATEGIES

PAHT is 100% preventable.[27] Comprehensive community-based programs may hold the key to successfully reducing morbidity and mortality from all forms of child maltreatment, including PAHT. Many programs have been developed to aid in this effort. Most are hospital based and focus on educating nurses and new parents. One such program was developed by the Worcester County Massachusetts Birthing Centers.[12] This program began by educating nurses on the dangers and warning signs of PAHT. The nurses were then trained to educate new parents and other caregivers using standardized curriculum and prepared materials.[12] A similar program was developed and implemented by the Norton Health Care Systems in Kentucky involving three hospitals.[28] Both programs work effectively for caregivers of newborns before hospital discharge.

EVIDENCE-BASED INTERVENTION

Recognizing that crying is the trigger most frequently identified by perpetrators of PAHT, the American Academy of Pediatrics in a 2009 policy statement recommended that pediatricians teach parents about the dangers of striking an infant's head or shaking an infant. Effective and safe strategies for coping with an infant's crying should be part of anticipatory guidance for parents and all infant caregivers.[7] Increasing a parent's awareness of the potential danger and understanding of normal crying patterns in infants can reduce the stress of dealing with a crying infant and reduce the child's risk of abuse.[27] Most birthing centers have incorporated some level of parental education related to crying into discharge planning. Reinforcing this teaching at a time when inconsolable crying is beginning to occur may prove to be an even more effective prevention strategy.

The Family Care Center Pediatric Clinic in Lexington, Kentucky, is a subsidiary of the University of Kentucky Health Care System. This clinic serves approximately 12,000 children annually. These families are primarily lower socioeconomic and at-risk. The clinic is staffed by pediatric nurse practitioners and serves as a training site for pediatric residents. With this diverse staff, the potential existed for a lack of consistency in providing family education on PAHT. One of the pediatric nurse practitioners, with support from the clinic's medical director, developed a comprehensive PAHT education program. The information is presented to all new parents at either the 2-week or the 1-month follow-up infant visit. To ensure consistency and quality it was determined that the clinic nurse was the best person to provide the established PAHT education to new parents. Several evidence-based PAHT prevention programs were evaluated for incorporation into the Clinic's PAHT educational protocol.

The Period of Purple Crying (**Box 1**), available from The National Center on Shaken Baby Syndrome, uses an acronym to help explain normal crying behaviors in infants. Also helpful is Dr Harvey Karp's five S's (shushing, side positioning, sucking, swaddling, and swinging).[27] Whatever structure is used infant caregivers need information on normal crying behaviors and specific strategies to deal with their personal stress related to infant crying.[27] See **Box 2** for more information.

Because every baby is not always a bundle of joy, parents should be provided with reasonable expectations. With this is mind, and using the best available information, the nurse at Family Care Center developed her own teaching materials. She used the acronym BUNDLE (**Box 3**) to teach parents about normal crying. Each letter serves as a reminder of one of six normal crying behaviors in the first 8 weeks of life. Parents are taught that *babies* cry often and *unexpectedly*. That sometimes *nothing* they do will sooth the baby and that the crying is often accompanied by a *distressed* look even when the baby is not in pain. They are told that the crying can *last* more than 5 hours daily and that it occurs more often in the *evening hours*. The parents are

---

Box 1
Period of Purple Crying

P	Peak of Crying: Your baby may cry more each day until he/she is about 8 weeks old
U	Unexpected: Crying can start and stop without any reason
R	Resist Soothing: Sometimes there is nothing you can do to make your baby stop crying
P	Pain-Like Face: When your baby cries he/she may look like they are in pain even when they are not.
L	Long Lasting: Crying episodes may last for 30–40 minutes or more. Some babies cry up to 5 hours a day.
E	Evening: More crying occurs in the late afternoon or evening

From National Center on Shaken Baby Syndrome, Period of PURPLE Crying program. Available at: http://www.dontshake.org/.

Box 2
Strategies for coping with a crying baby

What to do If Your Baby Won't Stop Crying

- Check on the baby. Make sure he/she isn't hungry and doesn't need a diaper change.
- Look for signs of illness like rash, swollen gums, or fever
- Offer a pacifier or toy to the baby
- Talk or sing to the baby
- Walk or rock the baby
- Take the baby for a car or stroller ride. Make sure he/she is safely strapped in a safety seat.
- Breathe slowly and calmly while holding the baby close against you.
- Ask for help. Take a break while a trustworthy relative or friend cares for the baby.
- When all else fails, place the baby safely on his/her back in the crib, close the door and take a 10-min break.
- See your child's health care provider to rule out a medical reason for the crying.

From KidsHealth.org. Abusive head trauma (shaken baby syndrome). 2011. Available at: http://kidshealth.org/parent/medical/brain/shaken.html#; with permission. This information was provided by KidsHealth®, one of the largest resources online for medically reviewed health information written for parents, kids, and teens. For more articles like this, visit KidsHealth.org or TeensHealth.org. © 1995–2013. The Nemours Foundation/KidsHealth®. All rights reserved.

---

also shown the video Portrait of Promise: Preventing Shaken Baby Syndrome, in which actual cases of PAHT are presented by victim's families. The video clearly demonstrates the devastating effects of shaking a baby. Parents are then given the opportunity to discuss the video and information given and to ask the nurse questions. A one-page informational sheet is also provided. This take-home message contains the definition of PAHT, some reasons why it occurs, the stress reduction techniques that were discussed at the visit, and local numbers that they can call for help or to ask questions. Also provided is information on what the caregiver should do if they suspect that their baby may have been shaken. Response to the program has been very positive.

CONCLUSIONS AND CLINICAL IMPLICATIONS

Nurses play a key role in the effort to reduce morbidity and mortality from all forms of child maltreatment, especially PAHT. Many states, such as Kentucky, which leads the nation in PAHT fatalities, have mandated continuing education on PAHT for all healthcare providers, including nurses.(28) Regardless of whether or not it is mandated by

---

Box 3
BUNDLE

B	Babies often cry more often each day for the first two months
U	Unexpected crying that comes and goes and you don't know why
N	No matter what you try your baby may continue to cry
D	Distressed look of pain, even when they're not
L	Lasting up to 5 hours or more a day
E	Evening hours is when your baby may cry the most

law every individual nurse can take steps to ensure that they are knowledgeable and effective in addressing issues of abuse with potential victims and families. An understanding of the consequences of abusive head trauma and the signs, symptoms, and patterns of injury commonly seen with abuse can reduce the chances that potential victims are missed. Nurses can also advocate for children by ensuring that comprehensive prevention programs are activated in their communities.

Nurses have a legal and a moral responsibility to intervene when they suspect that child abuse has occurred. Most states and territories of the United States have mandatory reporting laws that specifically address healthcare providers including nurses. It is not necessary that a nurse be able to prove that abuse has been or is occurring. A reasonable suspicion is enough to warrant a report. All nurses should keep a list of local, state, and national child abuse hotlines readily accessible. The national child abuse hotline is 1-800-4-A-CHILD. When making a report nurses should be objective and specific and give as many details as possible. Opinions are not facts and should never be offered.

Making the decision to file a report of suspected child abuse is not easy. Often there is no clear cut definitive proof that the injuries were deliberately inflicted. Nurses often have thoughts like "what if I am wrong and I cause this family all that trouble." Most nurses want to be liked by their patients and when suspecting abuse they worry about what the family will think of them if they file a report. It is especially difficult when the family presents with a loving concerned attitude. While preparing this article, one of this author's favorite patients (a 6 month old) presented with a bruise and an abrasion on the lobule of her ear (a cardinal warning sign for PAHT). The author had worked with this mother since the day after her baby was born and believed her to be a loving, caring mother. The decision to do a complete work-up for PAHT and to file a report of possible abuse was extremely difficult to make. Always remember that no matter how difficult reporting might be, the alternative could be a dead baby.

SUMMARY

PAHT is a significant cause of morbidity and mortality in the United States. Many infants and young children die from their injuries, whereas others sustain life-altering neurologic damage. Healthcare providers need to increase their knowledge base and level of suspicion when confronted with common vague presenting symptoms, such as vomiting, irritability, and feeding difficulties. Early recognition and appropriate action may significantly improve outcomes for victim of PAHT. Any provider who has reason to suspect abuse must take the necessary steps to protect the child. Comprehensive community-based programs that teach caregivers the dangers of shaking along with coping strategies for infant crying may hold the best hope of reducing the incidence of PAHT. Some communities choose to use available predeveloped materials, whereas others choose to develop their own materials. The important thing is that the information be disseminated to caregivers. Nurses can and should be leaders in this effort.

REFERENCES

1. Fang X, Brown DS, Florence CS, et al. The economic burden of child maltreatment in the United States and implications for prevention. Child Abuse Negl 2012. http://dx.doi.org/10.1016/j.chiabu.2011.10.006. Available at: http://www.sciencedirect.com/science/article/pii/S0145213411003140. Accessed July 6, 2012.
2. US Department of Health and Human Services, Administration for Children and Families, Administration on Children, Youth and Families, Children's Bureau. Child

Maltreatment 2009. Available at: http://www.acf.hhs.gov/programs/cb/stats_research/index.htm#can. Accessed August 12, 2012.

3. United States Government Accountability Office. Child maltreatment: strengthening national data on child fatalities could aid in prevention (GAO-11–599). 2011. Available at: http://www.gao.gov/new.items/d11599.pdf. Accessed July 6, 2012.

4. Centers for Disease Control and Prevention. Heads up: prevent shaken baby syndrome: it's not just a crime; it's a public health issue. Available at: http://www.cdc.gov/concussion/HeadsUp/sbs.html. Accessed July 6, 2012.

5. Parks SE, Annest JL, Hill HA, et al. Pediatric abusive head trauma: recommended definitions for public health surveillance and research. Atlanta (GA): Centers for Disease Control and Prevention; 2012.

6. Adamsbaum C, Grabar S, Mejean N, et al. Abusive head trauma: judicial admissions highlight violent and repetitive shaking. Pediatrics 2010;126:546.

7. Christian CW, Block R, Committee on Child Abuse and Neglect, American Academy of Pediatrics. Abusive head trauma in infants and children. Pediatrics 2009;123:1409–11.

8. Case ME, Graham MA, Handy TC, et al. Position paper on fatal abusive head injuries in infants and young children. Am J Forensic Med Pathol 2001;22:112.

9. Children Without a Voice USA. Abusive head trauma/SBS. 2012. Available at: http://www.childrenwithoutavoiceusa.org/cms/node/6. Accessed August 4, 2012.

10. US Department of Health and Human Services: Administration for Children and Families. Every Child Matters Education Fund. We can do better: child abuse and neglect deaths in the U.S. 2009. Available at: http://www.everychildmatters.org/about/issues/child-abuse-and-neglect. Accessed August 4, 2012.

11. Centers for Disease Control and Prevention, National Center for Injury Prevention and Control, Division of Violence Prevention. Shaken baby syndrome tip sheet. Available at: http://www.cdc.gov/healthmarketing/entertainment_education/tips/shaken_baby.htm. Accessed August 4, 2012.

12. Meskauskas L, Beaton K, Meservey M. Preventing shaken baby syndrome: a multidisciplinary response to six tragedies. Nurs Womens Health 2009;13(4):325–30.

13. Perlstein D. Shaken baby syndrome (SBS). 2008. Available at: http://www.medicinenet.com/script/main/art.asp?articlekey=92125&pf=3&page=1. Accessed August 11, 2010.

14. KidsHealth.org. Abusive head trauma (shaken baby syndrome). 2011. Available at: http://kidshealth.org/parent/medical/brain/shaken.html#a_What Are the Effects?. Accessed August 12, 2011.

15. Chiesa A, Duhaime C. Abusive head trauma. Pediatr Clin North Am 2009;56(2):317–31.

16. KidsHealth.org. Abusive head trauma (shaken baby syndrome). 2011. Available at: http://kidshealth.org/parent/medical/brain/shaken.html#a_How_These_Injuries_Happen. Accessed August 12, 2011.

17. Fulton DR. Shaken baby syndrome. Crit Care Nurs Q 2000;23(2):45–50.

18. MedlinePlus. Shaken baby syndrome. 2009. Available at: http://www.nlm.nih.gov/medlineplus/ency/article/000004.htm. Accessed July 5, 2012.

19. Esernio-Jenssen D, Tai J, Kodsi S. Abusive head trauma in children: a comparison of male and female perpetrators. Pediatrics 2001;127(4):649–57.

20. World Health Organization. Child maltreatment: fact sheet. 2010. Available at: http://www.who.int/mediacentre/factsheets/fs150/en/index.htm. Accessed August 1, 2012.

21. MedlinePlus. Child abuse rises when economy sags: study. 2012. Available at: http://www.nlm.nih.gov/medlineplus/news/fullstory_127270.html. Accessed August 12, 2012.
22. Ichord RN, Naim M, Pollock AN, et al. Hypox-ischemic injury complicates inflicted and accidental traumatic brain injury in young children: the role of diffusion-weighted imaging. J Neurotrauma 2007;24:106.
23. Geddes JF, Hackshaw AK, Vowles GH, et al. Neuropathology of inflected head injury in children. I. Patterns of brain damage. Brain 2001;124:1290.
24. Geddes JF, Vowles GH, Hackshaw AK, et al. Neuropathology of inflected head injury in children. II. Microscopic brain injury in infants. Brain 2001;124:1299.
25. Herman BE, Makoroff KL, Corneli HM. Abusive head trauma. Pediatr Emerg Care 2011;27(1):65–9.
26. Jenny C, Hymel KP, Ritzen A, et al. Abusive head trauma: an analysis of missed cases. JAMA 1999;281:621–6.
27. KidsHealth.org. Abusive head trauma (shaken baby syndrome). 2011. Available at: http://kidshealth.org/parent/medical/brain/shaken.html#a_Preventing AHT. Accessed May 12, 2011.
28. Gibbs J, Nevitt L. Strategies to reduce pediatric abusive head trauma in Kentucky: is parental education the key? J Obstet Gynecol Neonatal Nurs 2011;40:S27–8.

Childhood Bullying
A Review and Implications for Health Care Professionals

Vicki Hensley, MSN, APRN

KEYWORDS

- Bullying • Childhood bullying • Childhood violence • Bullying children

KEY POINTS

- Approximately 25% to 30% of children are affected by childhood bullying, either as a bully or as a victim.
- There are some common characteristics of bullies and victims. Knowing these will allow the health care provider to identify children at risk for or involved with bullying.
- Both bullies and victims have short- and long-term consequences of bullying.
- It is imperative that health care providers have knowledge about bullying.
- Health care providers need to take a pivotal role in assessing their patients for bullying and provide interventions as needed.

A teacher was teaching her class about bullying and gave them the following exercise to perform. She had the children take a piece of paper, crumble it up, stomp on it, and really mess it up, but be careful not to rip it. Then she had them unfold the paper, smooth it out, and look at how scarred and dirty it was. She then told them to tell it they were sorry. Now even though they said they were sorry and tried to fix the paper, she pointed out all the scars they had left behind. And that those scars would never go away no matter how hard they tried to fix it. That is what happens when a child bullies another child. They may say they are sorry but the scars are there forever.

—Anonymous.

BACKGROUND AND INTRODUCTION

Bullying is a widespread problem in our communities and schools that has perplexed school officials, teachers, parents, students, health care providers, and researchers for decades. Childhood bullying is certainly not a new concept; however, because

College of Nursing, University of Kentucky, 445 College of Nursing Building, 760 Rose Street, Lexington, KY 40536-0232, USA
E-mail address: Vrpack0@uky.edu

Nurs Clin N Am 48 (2013) 203–213
http://dx.doi.org/10.1016/j.cnur.2013.01.014
0029-6465/13/$ – see front matter Published by Elsevier Inc.
nursing.theclinics.com

of persistently high prevalence rates and the short- and long-term consequences of bullying, it is demanding more attention. It is normal child behavior to occasionally tease, play fight, and have disagreements with peers; however, bullying is a far more serious behavior that has short- and long-term academic, physical, and emotional effects on both the victim and the bully. It is crucial for nurses to be knowledgeable about bullying so that bullying can be assessed better and necessary interventions can be made available to those in need.

The purposes of this article are to describe bullying and the prevalence of bullying in the United States, discuss the common characteristics, including risk factors, of bullies and victims, discuss the short- and long-term consequences of bullying, and provide recommendations and considerations for assessing and intervening for bullying during childhood.

BULLYING OVERVIEW AND PREVALENCE

Bullying, which can be described in numerous ways, includes verbally, physically, and/or psychologically aggressive behavior that is intentionally harmful to another person and occurs repeatedly over time to an individual who is perceived to be less powerful physically and/or psychologically.[1] Bullying can involve physical overt behavior as well as verbal attacks, and nonverbal, nonphysical acts that are indirect and subtle. Obvious types of bullying include physical violence or threats, verbal abuse, and taunting or teasing, whereas less-obvious bullying can include social exclusion, manipulation of friendship, and negative text messages or Internet posts about someone. The most common form of bullying is verbal abuse and harassment, followed by social isolation and derogatory comments about physical appearance.[2] Bullying often occurs in an area with less adult supervision, such as bathrooms, playgrounds, cafeterias, and bus stops.[2] Often, bullies select someone who they perceive as different from themselves physically, emotionally, or intellectually. Bullying usually is a way for the bully to deal with their own problems. Bullies may also need to feel more superior to their peers or think bullying will gain them acceptance of their peers and make them feel more popular or important.[3]

Both boys and girls are involved in bullying others; however, there is conflicting evidence regarding the differences in bullying behavior between genders. Espelage and Swearer[4] caution against making definitive conclusions about gender differences in bullying. However, research does support that boys are more likely than girls to be bullies and are themselves also victimized by their peers. Girls are more likely to be victims of bullying during early adolescence.[5,6] The literature is more conclusive regarding age and ethnicity trends of bullying. Bullying increases for boys and girls during the late elementary years, peaks during middle school, and decreases in high school.[7] According to the US Department of Justice, Bureau of Justice Statistics' 2009 National Crime Victimization Survey: School Crime Supplement, students in higher grades were less likely to report bullying as compared with sixth graders. Students in sixth and seventh grade reported bullying the most and students in eighth grade were 50% less likely to report bullying, whereas 12th graders were 76% less likely to report bullying when compared with students in 6th and 7th grade.[8] There were no differences found in the prevalence of bullying by race or ethnicity.[8]

American children aged 8 to 15 years report that bullying is a greater problem than racism, pressure to have sexual intercourse, or use of alcohol and other drugs (Kaiser Family Foundation, 2001).[9] In a survey of over 5000 students in grades 7, 8, and 11 in an urban public school district, 26% of students were involved in bullying.[10] In another large study conducted by the National Institute of Child Health and Human

Development in 2009 of American students in grades 6 to 10, the magnitude of bullying was revealed by 37% of respondents having been victims of verbal harassment, 32% having been subjected to rumor spreading, 26% having experienced social isolation, 13% having been physically assaulted; and 10% having been cyberbullied.[11]

COMMON CHARACTERISTICS OF THE BULLY

There are common characteristics that bullies share. Bullies have aggressive attitudes toward their social encounters and a positive outlook about violence. Bullies are manipulative, need to dominate others, and lack empathy toward others. Bullies lack self-control and are guided by their impulses.[3,12] Children who bully others often come from a family in which aggression is modeled.[12] In a study involving 704 students aged 11 to 13 years, Viding and colleagues[13] concluded that those with higher callous and unemotional traits and conduct disorders were associated with higher levels of direct bullying.

Barboza and colleagues[14] examined the risk factors associated with bullying behavior of 9816 adolescents aged 11 to 14 years who completed a World Health Organization's Health Behavior in School-Aged Children Survey in 1997 to 1998. The investigators concluded that bullying increases among children who watch television frequently. Each standard deviation increase in hours of television watched per day increases the odds of being a bully by 21%, holding other variables constant.[14] Barboza and colleagues[14] also concluded that students who felt unsupported by their teachers, attended a school with an unfavorable environment, and had teachers and parents who did not place high expectations on their school performance were more likely to be a bully. Finally, students who had personally been a victim of bullying and felt emotional support from their peers were more likely to be a bully.[14] These results are well supported by other research studies.[3,15–17]

While there is significant literature describing bullying, several myths of bullying should be clarified. Bullies are not socially isolated. Research indicates bullies are at least somewhat popular and the more emotional support they receive regarding bullying, the more is bullying likely to occur.[1,3,14] Another common myth regarding bullying is bullies have low self-esteem. Research indicates bullies have average or above average self-esteem and are no more likely than their peers to be characterized as anxious or indecisive.[3,18] To effectively assess for bullying, nurses need to be cognizant of not only the common characteristics of bullies but also the common characteristics of students who are victims of bullying. The National Association of School Nurses (NASN) states that nurses must be able to identify those who bully and those who are at risk for or have experienced bullying.[19]

COMMON CHARACTERISTICS OF THE VICTIM

Like bullies, victims of bullying share several common characteristics. Victims of bullying are more anxious, depressed, insecure, and have low self-esteem when compared with other students.[13] Victims of bullying often lack friends at school and may be socially isolated. Children who are less physically attractive or overweight or who perform poorly in school are more likely to be bullied by others.[20] Children with disabilities such as cerebral palsy, autism, stammering, muscular dystrophy, or diabetes may also be more at risk of being a victim of bullying.[21] Victims of bullying are often described as not fitting in well with their peers. Shields and Cicchetti[22] surveyed 267 inner city children aged 8 to 12 years and concluded that children who had experienced maltreatment by a caregiver were more at risk of being bullied.

Perren and Alsaker[23] interviewed 345 children aged 5 to 7 years and their teachers regarding the children's social behavior, bullying, and victimization. The investigators concluded that victims were more submissive, had fewer leadership skills, were more withdrawn, were more isolated, were less cooperative, were less sociable, and frequently had no playmates.[23] Children who lack independence and maturity may also be subject to bullying.[24] Finnegan and colleagues[25] and Cohen and Canter[26] suggested that victimization was associated with those students who were perceived to have an overprotective parent. These students often fail to develop their own coping skills and are more likely to be bullied.

Children not only may bully others but also are victimized by their peers. These students are called bully/victims. Bully/victims demonstrate high levels of both aggression and depression and have lower academic scores, prosocial behavior, self-control, social acceptance, and self-esteem.[1,24,27,28] Veenstra and colleagues[29] analyzed the results of the Dutch TRacking Adolescents' Individual Lives Survey study that included 1065 adolescents. The investigators concluded that bully/victims were aggressive, had few friends and lower prosocial behavior, and were most disliked among students.[29] Perren and Alsaker[23] stated that bully/victims were less cooperative, less sociable, and more frequently had no playmates. Being informed about what characteristics a bully, victim, and bully/victim may possess will enable nurses and health care professionals to identify possible children at risk of bullying behavior and provide interventions that could reduce bullying and the consequences thereof.

CONSEQUENCES OF BULLYING

Bullying can have both short- and long-term academic, physical, and emotional consequences on both the bully and the victim. Being aware of the effects of bullying can allow nurses and health care providers to identify children who may be involved in bullying.

Short-Term Consequences

When children are involved in bullying behavior, they are more likely to report increased health-related problems including headaches, abdominal pain, anxiety, depression, and an increase in bed-wetting as well as other behavioral problems such as school avoidance, a decline in academic performance, poor relationships with peers, poor self-esteem, and loneliness.

Several studies have shown that victimization from bullying is associated with substantial adverse effects on physical and psychological health. In a cross-sectional study of 419 children in grades 1 to 10 by Lohre and colleagues[30] children reported emotional and somatic symptoms of sadness, anxiety, stomach aches, and headaches. Children's self-reported frequency of victimization was strongly and positively associated with their reports of emotional and somatic symptoms.[30] In another survey conducted by Farrow and Fox,[31] 376 adolescents completed self-report questionnaires on their experiences of bullying, emotional symptoms, and unhealthy eating and shape-related attitudes and behaviors. The findings suggest that the experience of bullying is positively correlated with depression and anxiety, restrained eating, and body dissatisfaction in both males and females.[31] Glew and colleagues[9] examined data collected from 3530 children in grades 3 to 5 and reported that both bullies and victims were more likely to report feeling unsafe at school and that they feel sad most days. Finally, Fekkes and colleagues[32] measured victimization from bullying as well as psychosocial and psychosomatic symptoms in 1118 children aged 9 to 11 years. The results of the study indicate that children who are victims of bullying have significantly higher chances of reporting psychosomatic and psychosocial problems, including depression, anxiety, bed-wetting, headaches, sleeping problems, abdominal pain, poor appetite, and feelings of tension or tiredness than children who were not bullied.[32]

When students are bullied on a regular basis, they may also experience homicidal or suicidal thoughts. The National Threat Assessment Center of the US Secret Service reviewed 37 school shootings and reported that more than two-thirds of the shooters felt "persecuted, threatened, attacked, or injured."[33]

Bullying behavior does not just affect the victim, but the bully suffers short-term consequences. According to the US Department of Justice, bullying is associated with vandalism, shoplifting, school absenteeism, dropping out of school, fighting, and drug and alcohol use.[34] Vernberg and colleagues[35] gathered data on 590 children in grades 3 to 5 by assessing victimization, aggression, and visits made to the school nurse. The results of the study suggest that involvement in bullying behavior as a bully or a victim is associated with increased somatic symptoms, illness, and injury complaints to the school nurse.[35] Hemphill and colleagues[36] analyzed the results of 5769 students who completed the International Youth Development Study. The investigators concluded that victimization of bullying was associated with an increased likelihood of depressive symptoms and bullying others was associated with an increased likelihood of theft, violent behavior, and binge drinking.

Long-Term Consequences

There are not only short-term consequences of being a bully or a victim of bullying but also long-term consequences that are evident into adult years of life. Numerous studies have shown that childhood bullying was associated with later violence, including criminal acts, alcohol and substance abuse, aggression, and antisocial behavior. Ragatz and colleagues[37] studied 960 college students who had reported being a bully, victim, or bully/victim during the last 2 years of high school and asked them about their current psychological characteristics and criminal behavior history. The investigators concluded that bullies and bully/victims had significantly higher scores on criminal thinking, psychopathy, and criminal behaviors than victims or controls. In addition, bully/victims tended to be male, were higher in criminal thinking, and had higher proactive aggression. In another study by Kim and colleagues[38] 957 participants were surveyed yearly from first or second grade up to the age of 21 years. It was concluded that childhood bullying was significantly associated with violence, heavy drinking, and marijuana use at the age of 21 years. Niemela and colleagues[39] found similar results in a study of 2946 children followed up from the age of 8 to 18 years. The investigators stated that bullying others frequently predicted illicit drug use. Furthermore, many researchers[40–47] have found childhood bullying to be positively correlated to subsequent criminal offending, including intimate partner violence, later in life. Olweus[45] states that former school bullies were heavily overrepresented in crime registers and 55% of those who bullied others during childhood had been convicted of one or more crimes by the time they were 24 years old.

Research on the long-term consequences of individuals who have been bullied show negative effects existing into adulthood and include greater risk for depression, anxiety, loneliness, posttraumatic stress, and problems with interpersonal functioning. In the study conducted by Niemela and colleagues[39] as described earlier, researchers concluded that victims were associated with a lower occurrence of illicit drug use; however, victimization may predispose a child to subsequent smoking. Olweus[48] reported that individuals who were bullied during childhood were more likely to be depressed and have poorer self-esteem at the age of 23 years than nonvictimized adults. In another study conducted by Jantzer and colleagues[49] of 170 college students, it was concluded that victimization was positively correlated with contemporaneous shyness levels and was negatively correlated with friendship quality and trust. Finally, in 2005, Newman and colleagues[50] surveyed 853 undergraduate college students asking about their bullied experiences, their reactions to them, and their current emotional state. The researchers reported that those who were bullied during childhood had higher levels of stress and felt more isolated than nonvictimized adults.[50]

Therefore, bullying not only remains a serious threat to children's physical and emotional health during the time they are involved in bullying behavior but also may be an indicator of serious psychiatric, behavior, and psychosocial symptoms and problems that can persist for many years into adulthood.

GUIDELINES

The role of the pediatric health care provider regarding bullying assessment, intervention, and prevention is well recognized by many professional organizations, including the American Academy of Pediatrics (AAP). The AAP states that pediatric health care providers can contribute to bullying prevention through promotion of strong parenting skills and recognition, screening, and appropriate referrals of patients involved in bullying behaviors.[51]

The Society for Adolescent Medicine emphasizes that pediatric health care providers should be familiar with the characteristics of youth possibly involved with bullying, sensitive to signs and symptoms of bullying and victimization, and intervene when necessary.[52] Srabstein, the medical director for the Clinic for Health Problems Related to Bullying at Children's National Medical Center, states pediatric health care providers must take the time to ask patients if they are being bullied or if they are bullying others.[53] The National Center for Mental Health Promotion and Youth Violence Prevention states that bullying is best addressed by comprehensive approach and health care professionals can play a large role in preventing bullying by taking opportunities, including wellness examinations, to assess children for signs of bullying.[54]

The NASN states school nurses need to have the skills to assess students for bullying behavior as well as to identify characteristics of both victims and bullies.[19] By being knowledgeable about bullying, those at risk of bullying, and the consequences of bullying, school nurses will be readily able to identify potential students involved with bullying, assess for bullying in these students, and intervene with effective bullying prevention strategies.

NURSING IMPLICATIONS

Nurses are in a unique position to identify potential students at risk of either bullying others or being a victim of bullying and provide interventions to the child, which can reduce the prevalence of bullying behaviors. Everyday nurses assess children for a variety of problems and potential threats to their health. School nurses may be the first to identify students at risk or involved in bullying behaviors. These nurses are in a prime location to assess for bullying and provide interventions for those in need. In a survey of 404 school nurses, Hendershot and colleagues[55] reported that 80% would assess and document injuries and refer to the principle, 77% would refer the students to the school counselor, 74% would make the teachers and staff aware of the situation, 71% would talk to the bully, and 45% would work with the victim about ways to avoid bullying. School nurses also reported that they felt that effective ways of dealing with bullying included improving supervision, using bullying prevention techniques, assisting students with warning signs of bullying, and implementing bullying response activities.[55]

Victimization causes an increase in health-related symptoms, such as headaches, abdominal pain, anxiety, and depression. When health care providers see clients with these ailments, the practitioner should be cognizant that bullying could be contributing to these issues and ask the patient if anyone is bullying them. Health care providers should also routinely screen their patients for bullying behavior. The well-child examination may provide an opportunistic time in which to ask patients if they bully others or are being bullied by someone else. When bullying behaviors are confirmed, the health care provider can provide many interventions to the patient, including management of the behavior, whether it is bullying others or victimization, and this is best done through a multidisciplinary effort involving parents, teachers, school counselors and administrators, and mental health professionals. The health care provider should provide education and support for the patient and family, help parents locate and use resources regarding bullying, refer the patient for counseling if needed, and secure help from the child's school to help stop the bullying behavior.

To foster the assessment of bullying, the health care provider should have a list of simple direct questions to ask the child and parent. Sample questions are included in **Box 1**. These questions can provide the health care provider with insight regarding whether the child has been bullied or is involved with bullying behaviors.

RESEARCH IMPLICATIONS

Given the high number of children who are bullied and the lack of effective interventions to reduce bullying behavior, additional research is needed regarding childhood bullying. Research targeting health care professionals and assessing their current beliefs and practices regarding bullying assessment and interventions would provide the foundation for further intervention studies regarding health care providers addressing bullying behaviors. A survey instrument used by health care providers

---

Box 1
Example questions to use for assessment of bullying

Questions for child

1. Have you ever been teased or picked on by other students at school?
2. At recess do you usually play with other children or by yourself?
3. Do you sometimes dread going to school or are you afraid to go to school?
4. Have you called another student names or made fun of them?
5. Have you hurt another student on purpose?
6. Have you ever stopped another student from playing with you or joining your group during play time?

Questions for parents

1. Does your child frequently complain of headaches or belly pains, is frequently sad, or tries to avoid going to school?
2. Do you have any concerns that your child is having problems with other children at school?
3. Who are some of your child's friends at school?
4. Has your child ever told you he/she was being picked on or bullied at school?

during well-child examinations or by the school nurse would be an effective method to assess for bullying. The instrument would need to be easily administered and scored.

Other areas of research are needed to test appropriate interventions that health care providers can use regarding bullying reduction and prevention. Research focusing on students who are bully/victims is also important to facilitate better understanding of this phenomenon and the consequences. Longitudinal studies would also be helpful in understanding the long-term implications of being a bully, and because the research is minimal, of being bullied and being a bully/victim. Last, studies involving the relationship between victimization and psychosocial and health-related symptoms would provide insight into potential interventions to help protect these individuals and reduce the consequences of bullying.

SUMMARY

Childhood bullying is a well-documented problem associated with many short- and long-term consequences. Even though there is much literature about the phenomenon, the issue continues to be unresolved and problematic for children. It is imperative that health care professionals, including pediatricians, nurse practitioners, physician assistants, and nurses alike, be knowledgeable about the multidimensional nature of bullying and begin assessing children for this type of violence. Direct questions about being bullied should be asked at each well-child visit as well as at acute visits where children present with symptoms that could be caused by bullying. Questioning will not only identify if problems exist but also allow for dialogue to happen between the child and the parent. Furthermore, questioning will also identify those patients who need interventions to help reduce the consequences of bullying behavior.

REFERENCES

1. Nansel TR, Overpeck M, Pilla RS, et al. Bullying behaviors among US youth: prevalence and association with psychosocial adjustment. JAMA 2001;285(16): 2094–100.
2. Shellard E. Recognizing and preventing bullying. The informed educator series. Arlington (VA): Educational Research Service; 2002.
3. Aleude O, Adeleke F, Omoike D, et al. A review of the extent, nature, characteristics and effects of bullying behavior in schools. J Instr Psychol 2008;35(2):151–8.
4. Espelage DL, Swearer SM. Gender differences in bullying: moving beyond mean level differences. In: Espelage DL, Swearer SM, editors. Bullying in American schools: a social-ecological perspective on prevention and intervention. Mahwah (NJ): Erlbaum; 2004. p. 15–35.
5. Olweus D. Bullying at school: what we know and what we can do. Cambridge (MA): Blackwell Publishing, Inc; 1993.
6. Kim YS, Boyce WT, Koh YJ, et al. Time trends, trajectories, and demographic predictors of bullying: a prospective study in Korean adolescents. J Adolesc Health 2009;45(4):360–7.
7. Garrett AG. Bullying in American schools. Jefferson (NC): McFarland; 2003.
8. U.S. Department of Justice, Office of Justice Programs, Bureau of Justice Statistics. National crime victimization survey school crime supplement, 2009 [Codebook]. Ann Arbor (MI): Interuniversity Consortium for Political and Social Research; 2009.
9. Kaiser Family Foundation and Children Now. Bullying, discrimination and sexual pressures "Big Problems" for today's tweens and younger kids; parents often wait

for their kids to raise tough issues. 2001. Available at: http://www.kff.org/mediapartnerships/3105-index.cfm. Accessed August 25, 2012.

10. Glew GM, Fan MY, Katon W, et al. Bullying and school safety. J Pediatr 2008; 152(1):123–8.

11. Wang J, Iannotti RJ, Nansel TR. School bullying among US adolescents: physical, verbal, relational, and cyber. J Adolesc Health 2009;45(4):368–75.

12. Carter S. Bullies and power: a look at the research. Issues Compr Pediatr Nurs 2011;34:97–102.

13. Viding E, Simmonds E, Petrides K, et al. The contribution of callous-unemotional traits and conduct problems to bullying in early adolescence. J Child Psychol Psychiatry 2009;50(4):471–81.

14. Barboza GE, Schiamberg LB, Oehmke J, et al. Individual characteristics and the multiple contexts of adolescent bullying: an ecological perspective. J Youth Adolesc 2009;38:101–21.

15. Espelage DL, Bosworth K, Simon TR. Examining the social context of bullying behaviors in early adolescence. J Couns Dev 2000;78(3):326–33.

16. Duffy AL, Nesdale D. Peer groups, social identity, and children's bullying behavior. Soc Dev 2008;18:121–39.

17. Olweus D, Limber S, Mihalic S. Blueprints for violence prevention, book nine: bullying prevention program. Boulder (CO): Center for the Study and Prevention of Violence; 1999.

18. O'Moore M, Kirkham C. Self-esteem and its relationships to bullying behaviour. Aggress Behav 2001;27:269–83.

19. National Association of School Nurses (NASN). Peer bullying. 2003. Available at: http://www.nasn.org. Accessed August 19, 2011.

20. Sweeting H, West P. Being different: correlates of the experience of teasing and bullying at age 11. Res Paper Educ 2001;16(3):225–46.

21. Storch E, Lwein A, Silverstein J, et al. Social-psychological correlates of peer victimization in children with endocrine disorders. J Pediatr 2004;145(6):784.

22. Shields A, Cicchetti D. Parental maltreatment and emotion dysregulation as risk factors for bullying and victimization in middle childhood. J Clin Child Psychol 2001;30:349–63.

23. Parren S, Alsaker FD. Social behavior and peer relationships of victims, bully-victims, and bullies in kindergarten. J Child Psychol Psychiatry 2006;47(1):45–57.

24. Nansel TR, Overpeck W, Overpeck MD, et al. Cross-national consistency in the relationship between bullying behaviors and psychosocial adjustment. Arch Pediatr Adolesc Med 2004;158:730–6.

25. Finnegan RA, Hodges EV, Perry DG. Victimization by peers: associations with children's reports of mother-child interaction. J Pers Soc Psychol 1998;75: 1076–86.

26. Cohen A, Canter A. Bullying: facts for schools and parents. National Association of School Psychologists. 2003. Available at: http://naspcenter.org. Accessed August 19, 2011.

27. Hanish LD, Guerra NG. Aggressive victims, passive victims, and bullies: developmental continuity or developmental change? Merrill-Palmer Quarterly 2004; 50:17–38.

28. Schwartz D. Subtypes of victims and aggressors in children's peer groups. J Abnorm Child Psychol 2000;28:181–92.

29. Veenstra R, Lindenberg S, Oldehinkel AJ, et al. Bullying and victimization in elementary schools: a comparison of bullies, victims, bully/victims, and uninvolved preadolescents. Dev Psychol 2005;41(4):672–82.

30. Lohre A, Lyderson ST, Paulsen B, et al. Peer victimization as reported by children, teachers, and parents in relation to children's health symptoms. BMC Public Health 2011;11:278.
31. Farrow CV, Fox CL. Gender differences in the relationships between bullying at school and healthy eating and shape-related attitudes and behaviors. Br J Educ Psychol 2011;81:409–20.
32. Fekkes M, Pijpers FI, Fredriks M, et al. Do bullied children get ill, or do ill children get bullied? A prospective cohort study on the relationship between bullying and health-related symptoms. Pediatrics 2006;117:1568–74.
33. Vossekuil B, Reddy M, Fein R, et al. Safe school initiative: an interim report on the prevention of targeted violence in schools. U.S. Secret Service National Threat Assessment Center in collaboration with the U.S. Department of education and with support from the National Institute of Justice. 2000.
34. U.S. Department of Justice, Office of Justice Programs. Addressing the problem of juvenile bullying. OJJDP Fact Sheet. 2001. Available at: https://www.ncjrs.gov/pdffiles1/ojjdp/FS200127.pdf. Accessed August 19, 2011.
35. Vernberg EM, Nelson TD, Fonagy P, et al. Victimization, aggression, and visits to the school nurse for somatic complaints, illnesses, and physical injuries. Pediatrics 2011;127(5):842–8.
36. Hemphill SA, Kotevski A, Herrenkohl TI, et al. Longitudinal consequences of adolescent bullying perpetration and victimization: a study of students in Victoria, Australia. Crim Behav Ment Health 2011;21:107–16.
37. Ragatz LL, Anderson RJ, Fremouw W, et al. Criminal thinking patterns, aggression styles, and the psychopathic traits of late high school bullies and bully-victims. Aggress Behav 2011;37:145–60.
38. Kim MJ, Catalano RF, Haggerty KP, et al. Bullying at elementary school and problem behavior in young adulthood: a study of bullying, violence and substance use from age 11 to age 21. Crim Behav Ment Health 2011;21:136–44.
39. Niemela S, Brunstein-Klomek A, Sillanmaki L, et al. Childhood bullying behaviors at age eight and substance use at age 18 among males. A nationwide prospective study. Addict Behav 2011;36:256–60.
40. Sourander A, Jensen P, Ronning JA, et al. Childhood bullies and victims and their risk of criminality in late adolescence. Arch Pediatr Adolesc Med 2007;161:546–52.
41. Falb KL, McCauley HL, Decker MR, et al. School bullying perpetration and other childhood risk factors as predictors of adult intimate partner violence perpetration. Arch Pediatr Adolesc Med 2011;165(10):890–4.
42. Bender D, Losel F. Bullying at school as a predictor of delinquency, violence and other anti-social behavior in adulthood. Crim Behav Ment Health 2011;21:99–106.
43. Farrington DP, Ttofi MM. Bullying as a predictor of offending violence and later life outcomes. Crim Behav Ment Health 2011;21:90–8.
44. Jiang D, Walsh M, Augimeri LK. The linkage between childhood bullying behavior and future offending. Crim Behav Ment Health 2011;21:128–35.
45. Olweus D. Bullying at school and later criminality: findings from three Swedish community samples of males. Crim Behav Ment Health 2011;21:151–6.
46. Renda J, Vassallo S, Edwards B. Bullying in early adolescence and its association with anti-social behavior, criminality and violence 6 and 10 years later. Crim Behav Ment Health 2011;21:117–27.
47. Ttofi MM, Farrington DP, Losel F, et al. The predictive efficiency of school bullying verses later offending: a systematic/meta-analytic review of longitudinal studies. Crim Behav Ment Health 2011;21:80–9.

48. Olweus D. Bullying at school: long-term outcomes for the victims and an effective school-based intervention program. In: Huesmann LR, editor. Aggressive behavior: current perspectives. New York: Plenum Press; 1994. p. 97–130.
49. Jantzer AM, Hoover JH, Narloch R. The relationship between school-aged bullying and trust, shyness, and quality of friendships in young adulthood: a preliminary research note. Sch Psychol Int 2006;27:146–56.
50. Newman ML, Holden GW, Delville Y. Isolation and the stress of being bullied. J Adolesc 2005;28:343–57.
51. Committee on Injury, Violence, and Poison Prevention. Role of the pediatrician in youth violence prevention. Pediatrics 2009;124:393–402.
52. Eisenberg ME, Aalsma MC. Bullying and peer victimization: position paper of the Society for Adolescent Medicine. J Adolesc Health 2005;36(1):88–91.
53. Infectious Diseases in Children. Bullying: what a pediatrician should know. 2011. Available at: http://www.healio.com/Pediatrics/news/print. Accessed August 25, 2012.
54. National Center for Mental Health Promotion and Youth Violence Prevention. Available at: http://www.promoteprevent.org/publications/prevention-briefs/preventing-bullying-schools-and-community. Accessed August 25, 2012.
55. Hendershot C, Dake JA, Price JH, et al. Elementary school nurses' perceptions of student bullying. J Sch Nurs 2006;22(4):229–36.

College Sorority Members' Knowledge and Behaviors Regarding Human Papillomavirus and Cervical Cancer

Mollie E. Aleshire, DNP, FNP-BC, PNP-BC[a],*, Sharon E. Lock, PhD, APRN[b],
Lynne A. Jensen, PhD, APRN[c]

KEYWORDS

- Human papillomavirus • Cervical cancer • College students • Knowledge • Behavior
- Vaccination

KEY POINTS

- Human papillomavirus (HPV) is most prevalent in college-age youth.
- Unhealthy sexual behaviors continue to be a major risk factor for morbidity in adolescents and young people.
- Education about sexual health, vaccination for HPV, and screening for cervical cancer can help prevent HPV and its sequelae.
- Health care providers must not only educate clients about HPV and cervical cancer, but must also actively recommend vaccination against HPV as the most effective prevention strategy for HPV and cervical cancer.

BACKGROUND AND SIGNIFICANCE

Prevalence of HPV and Cervical Cancer

The incidence of genital human papillomavirus (HPV) is higher in female college students than in many other populations. Young people aged 15 to 24 years acquire nearly one-half of all new sexually transmitted diseases (STDs). Cervical HPV is the most common STD in college-age women.[1–3] Seventy-four percent of new HPV infections occur in those aged 15 to 24 with peak prevalence worldwide in females 25 years or younger.[4–6] In 2000, it was estimated that some 9.2 million 15- to 24-year-olds in the

---

The authors have nothing to disclose.
[a] College of Nursing, University of Kentucky, 450A CON Building, Lexington, KY 40536-0232, USA; [b] College of Nursing, University of Kentucky, 563 CON Building, Lexington, KY 40536-0232, USA; [c] College of Nursing, University of Kentucky, 450E CON Building, Lexington, KY 40536-0232, USA
* Corresponding author.
E-mail address: mollie.aleshire@uky.edu

United States were infected with HPV.[1] The National Health and Nutrition Examination Survey (NHANES) showed HPV prevalence among females was highest from 20 to 24 years. The HPV prevalence among sexually active females aged 14 to 19 years was approximately 33% and increased to 53.8% among sexually active females aged 20 to 24.[3,7] The purpose of this study is to discover female college sorority members' knowledge and knowledge gaps regarding HPV and cervical cancer, to identify sexual and health behaviors in this group, and to determine whether there is any relationship between HPV/cervical cancer knowledge and sexual/health behaviors in this population.

Despite the fact that genital HPV infection and other STDs are increasingly common among young, sexually active women, unhealthy sexual behaviors continue to be a major risk factor for morbidity in college students.[8] The American College Health Association (ACHA) National College Health Assessment in Fall 2011 surveyed 27,774 college students at 44 postsecondary institutions in the United States.[8] Within the past 30 days of taking the survey, 49% of female students and 42.9% of male students reported having vaginal sex, 41.5% of female students and 41.4% of male students reported having oral sex, and 4.7% of female students and 6% of male students reported having anal sex. In the previous 12 months, 45.9% of female students and 40.5% of male students reported having 1 sexual partner, with 22.1% females and 26.2 males having more than 1 partner. For those students who had been sexually active in the previous 30 days, 48.6% of females and 55.5% of males reported using a condom mostly or always with vaginal intercourse. With anal intercourse 22.1% of females and 35.5% of males used condoms, and only 5.4% of females and 4.9% of males used condoms with oral sex.[8]

HPV infection has been firmly established as the primary cause of cervical cancer.[9] HPV infections also have been shown to lead to carcinomas at other sites and to genital condylomata.[7] HPV infections are now the most common STDs among sexually active populations worldwide.[10] HPV DNA is present in 99.7% of women with histologically confirmed squamous cell cervical cancer.[11]

An investigation found the overall prevalence of HPV infection among females aged 14 to 59 years in the United States to be 26.8%.[7] Three out of every 4 individuals of reproductive age in the United States have been infected with genital strains of HPV. Annually in the United States there are an estimated 6.2 million new HPV infections, and the estimated prevalence of HPV is approximately 20 million. It is estimated that 80% of sexually active women will have been infected with HPV by the time they are 50 years old.[12] Infection with HPV type 16 accounts for about half of cervical cancers worldwide, and HPV type 16 seroprevalence in women aged 12 to 59 years in the United States is approximately 17.9%.[13] The United States spends approximately 4 billion dollars annually to manage the consequences of HPV infections, specifically abnormal cervical changes and cancer.[12]

Cervical cancer is the second most common cancer in women worldwide[14] and remains a major cause of morbidity and mortality among women in the United States.[15] Worldwide, the estimated burden of disease from cervical cancer from 2002 to 2005 was 274,000 annual deaths and 3.3 million disability-adjusted life years lost.[16–18] Every year approximately 12,000 women in the United States are diagnosed with cervical cancer and more than 3000 women will die as a result of the disease.[19] Alarmingly, cervical cancer remains one of the top 10 cancer sites for African American, Hispanic, American Indian, and Alaska Native females in the United States,[15] this despite available access for most women to the Papanicolaou (Pap) test,[20] which the United States Preventive Services Task Force (USPSTF) (2009) cites as the most effective method of screening for cervical cancer in sexually active females.[21]

Several risk factors associated with HPV infection in young adult women have been identified: age 25 to 30 years, lack of condom use with intercourse, history of an STD other than HPV, a sexual partner more than 2 years older, more than 3 lifetime sexual partners, a new sexual partner in the last 12 months, illegal drug use, sexual activity while impaired by alcohol, and never being married.[15,22,23]

Knowledge of HPV and Cervical Cancer

In the United States, knowledge of HPV tends to be poor. In research by Benning and Lund,[24] only 43% of the women surveyed had heard of HPV. Even women who had previously had an abnormal Pap smear were no more likely to have heard of HPV or to know that HPV is the primary cause of cervical cancer than those who had not had an abnormal Pap smear.[24] University students also have scant HPV knowledge. Yacobi and colleagues[25] found that only 37% of their survey respondents had heard of HPV, and the median score (range 0–14) regarding HPV knowledge and awareness was 3. Of 7 STDs assessed, the students knew the least about HPV.

Wong and Sam[2] assessed knowledge of HPV and cervical cancer in an ethnically diverse female college student population, and the mean knowledge score (range 0–14) across their sample was only 3.25. Female nursing students, African American college students, and Latina college students are other populations that also have been shown to lack HPV knowledge and awareness.[26,27]

Scant research has examined the relationship between sexual/health behaviors in female college students and knowledge of HPV and cervical cancer. Ingledue and colleagues[28] found that college women exhibit high-risk sexual behaviors, but low knowledge level related to HPV. Most of the students in the study were in a sexual relationship, with 25% of respondents reporting 2 or more sexual partners within the past year. Nearly half of the students reported inconsistent condom use (less than 50% of the time), whereas only 15% of survey participants indicated they always used condoms. Forty-eight percent of these young women used oral contraceptives, 20% smoked cigarettes, and nearly one-fourth of these female students had never had a Pap test. The average knowledge score (range 0–15) was 6.8 with a standard deviation of 3.6. No significant relationships were found between HPV/cervical cancer knowledge and number of sexual partners or condom use. However, those who were more knowledgable regarding HPV/cervical cancer were more likely to have had a Pap test in the past year.[28]

Denny-Smith and colleagues[27] found that female nursing students' average knowledge score was 10.2 (range 0–15) when surveyed regarding HPV/cervical cancer. Nearly three-fourths of these students were involved in a sexual relationship, with the majority (67.9%) reporting 1 sexual partner in the past year. More than 60% of these female students reported condom use occasionally or less. Most of the respondents did not smoke cigarettes. Forty percent were using oral contraceptives, and most reported having a Pap smear in the last year. There were no significant relationships between HPV/cervical cancer knowledge and condom use. However, these researchers found that as HPV/cervical cancer knowledge increased, so did the number of sexual partners in this group. Moreover, those with more knowledge of HPV/cervical cancer were more likely to have had a Pap smear in the last year.[27]

No research has been identified in determining whether HPV/cervical cancer knowledge has any relationship to sexual and health behaviors in college female sorority members. Sorority members have been shown to be more likely than their nonsorority peers to have unprotected sex after drinking and to have not used a condom during vaginal intercourse. Sorority members are also less likely than their fraternity counterparts to have used a condom during vaginal intercourse.[29] Knowledge of HPV/cervical cancer by sorority members is important because sorority members have been shown to influence their peers, both sorority and nonsorority college students.[30] Although cervical cancer often develops later in life, most HPV infections occur in the age group of most college students.

Prevention of HPV and Cervical Cancer

In 2006 the US Food and Drug Administration approved the use of the quadrivalent HPV vaccine for females aged 9 to 26 years, which was followed by the Centers for Disease Control and Prevention (CDC) Advisory Committee on Immunization Practices (ACIP) 2007 recommendation that females aged 11 to 12 routinely receive HPV vaccination and that young women aged 13 to 26 receive catch-up HPV vaccination. Approximately 49% of female teens have started the 3 vaccine series to prevent HPV, but only 32% of teenage girls have received the recommended 3 doses of the HPV vaccine.[19] College females need to have knowledge of HPV and its sequelae to positively influence the decision to be vaccinated against HPV. The goal of increased HPV vaccination is to ultimately decrease HPV incidence and prevalence.

METHODS
Design

This study used a quantitative, nonexperimental, descriptive design. Knowledge of HPV and cervical cancer, and health behaviors of female sorority members, were evaluated. Relationships between HPV and cervical cancer knowledge and sexual and health behaviors in this group were also assessed.

Participants

Study participants were a convenience sample of female college sorority members at a large, southern, public university. Criteria for inclusion in the study included female gender, sorority membership at the university where the study was conducted, age 18 to 25 years, ability to read and comprehend the English language, and an e-mail address on file with the university office of Fraternity and Sorority Affairs.

The Assistant Dean of Students, who is also the Director of Fraternity and Sorority Affairs, agreed to encourage and facilitate study participation by university sorority members and provided sorority members' e-mail addresses to the investigator. The study was granted approval by the university Institutional Review Board with an exemption for signed consent. The proposed study was also reviewed and approved by the National Panhellenic Council Research Committee before implementation.

Two hundred forty-eight female sorority members voluntarily participated in the research. The respondents' ages ranged from 18 to 22 years, and all were single.

Instrument

The instrument was a survey titled Awareness of HPV and Cervical Cancer Questionnaire, which has been used in previous research.[27,28] Permission to use and modify the survey was granted by the survey's author. The original 40-item questionnaire was developed by Ingledue and colleagues[28] to assess knowledge, perceptions, and sexual risk behaviors related to HPV and cervical cancer. Ingledue and colleagues reported high reliability using test-retest methods over a 2-week period (knowledge = 0.90; behaviors = 0 .90), and established the instrument's content validity via a panel of experts.

The knowledge and behavior portions of the survey were used for this research study (**Box 1** lists the items). Questions 1 to 15 were the knowledge questions of

Box 1
Questionnaire

Choose 1 answer for each of the following:

1. The virus associated with cervical cancer is transmitted by: a. Sexual intercourse, b. Maternal-fetal transmission, c. Blood transfusions, d. Inanimate objects

2. Cervical cancer and precancer cells are associated with the presence of: a. Epstein-Barr virus, b. Herpes simplex virus, c. Human papillomavirus, d. Human immune deficiency virus

3. Cervical cancer can be diagnosed by: a. X-ray, b. Pap tests, c. Blood tests, d. Urine tests

4. Prevention of cervical cancer may require: a. Delayed onset of sexual activity, b. Annual Pap test, c. Use of condoms, d. All of the above

5. Human papillomavirus (HPV) can cause: a. Vaginal discharge, b. Genital warts, c. Itching, d. Burning urination

6. Human papillomavirus (HPV) can live in the skin without causing growths or changes? a. Yes, b. No

7. Having multiple sex partners is a risk factor for cervical cancer? a. Yes, b. No

8. Having genital warts is a risk factor for cervical cancer? a. Yes, b. No

9. Having sexual intercourse before age 18 is a risk factor for cervical cancer? a. Yes, b. No

10. Taking illegal drugs is a risk factor for cervical cancer? a. Yes, b. No

11. Having contracted any sexually transmitted diseases is a risk factor for cervical cancer? a. Yes, b. No

12. Smoking cigarettes is a risk factor for cervical cancer? a. Yes, b. No

13. Poor diet or nutrition is a risk factor for cervical cancer? a. Yes, b. No

14. Using tampons is a risk factor for cervical cancer? a. Yes, b. No

15. Use of oral contraceptives is a risk factor for cervical cancer? a. Yes, b. No

16. How old are you? a. Younger than 18, b. 18, c. 19, d. 20, e. 21, f. 22, g. 23, h. 24, i. 25, j. Older than 25

17. What is your sexual status? a. Currently involved in a sexual relationship, b. Have had sexual intercourse but not currently involved in a sexual relationship, c. Never had sexual intercourse

18. What is the number of sexual partners that you have had within the past year? a. 0, b. 1, c. 2, d. 3, e. 4, f. 5, g. 6, h. 7, i. 8, j. 9. k. 10, l. >10

19. Do you use condoms? a. Always (100% of time), b. Usually (76%–99% of time), c. Sometimes (51%–75% of time), d. Occasionally (26%–50% of time), e. Rarely (1%–25% of time), f. Never (0% of time)

20. Do you currently use oral contraceptives? a. Yes, b. No

21. Do you currently smoke cigarettes? a. Yes, b. No

22. What is your marital status? a. Single, b. Married

23. When was the last time you had a Pap test? a. Never, b. Within the past year, c. Have had one but not in the past year

24. Has you or anyone in your family ever been diagnosed with human papillomavirus (HPV) or cervical cancer? a. Yes, b. No

Adapted from Ingledue K, Cottrell R, Bernard A. College women's knowledge, perceptions, and preventive behaviors regarding human papillomavirus infection and cervical cancer. Am J Health Stud 2004;19(1):28–34; with permission.

the survey, consisting of multiple-choice questions with only 1 correct answer. Correct answers were scored as 1 while incorrect answers received a score of 0. Thus the possible range of scores was from 0 to 15, with higher scores indicating higher knowledge levels. Questions 16 to 24 were multiple-choice questions addressing demographics and sexual risk behaviors.

Data Collection

E-mails were sent to 2220 female sorority members. The e-mails contained a detailed letter explaining the research project, detailing the voluntary nature of participation, and assuring participant anonymity. Participants electing to take part in the research could then click onto a link in thetaking them directly to the survey, which was available via SurveyMonkey. SurveyMonkey only collected item responses without any record of any identifying data.

Data Analysis

Data results were analyzed using SPSS 14.0 for Windows Student Version. Descriptive statistical analysis was used to describe participant demographics and behavioral profile. Analysis of variance (ANOVA) was computed to determine mean differences in knowledge scores. Relationships between HPV/cervical cancer knowledge and condom use as well as relationships between knowledge and the number of sexual partners within the last year were determined using the Spearman rank correlation. Differences in knowledge scores for those using condoms, smokers, and family diagnosis of cervical cancer were analyzed using t-tests.

RESULTS

Two hundred forty-eight students completed surveys for an 11.2% response rate. All participants ranged in age from 18 to 22 years with a relatively normal distribution. The average age of respondents was 20 years. None of the sorority members were married.

Descriptive statistical analysis helped develop an overall behavioral profile for this group of sorority students (**Table 1**). Sexual status had a relatively even distribution, with approximately one-third of sorority females in a current sexual relationship, one-third in no current sexual relationship, and a third who indicated they had never had sexual intercourse. Many (65%) research participants indicated having only 1 or no sexual partners in the last year. Condom use varied quite widely among the 248 sorority respondents. Over half of this group used condoms 75% of the time or more, but a quarter of these students used condoms 50% of the time or less. Slightly more than half (54.8%) were using oral contraceptives. The majority (91.9%) of these sorority students did not smoke cigarettes. Pap tests had been completed within the last year by 62% of this group. Twenty-one percent of these women indicated a personal or family medical history of HPV or cervical cancer.

Knowledge scores had a possible range of 0 to 15 for each individual, with higher scores showing greater knowledge related to HPV and cervical cancer. The range of scores was 4 to 15, with a mean knowledge score of 10.72 and a standard deviation of 2.00. The most frequent knowledge score (mode) was 10. More than 90% of survey participants knew that the virus associated with cervical cancer is transmitted by sexual intercourse, that cervical cancer and precancer cells are associated with the presence of HPV, and that Pap tests can aid in the diagnosis of cervical cancer. Knowledge regarding behaviors to aid in the prevention of cervical cancer was also high. Nearly all participants knew that HPV can live in the skin without causing growths

Table 1 Descriptive data and health-related behaviors (N = 248)		
Characteristics	**n**	**%**
Age (y)		
18	45	18.1
19	61	24.6
20	67	27.0
21	56	22.6
22	18	7.3
Sexual experience status		
Current sexual relationship	97	39.1
No current sexual relationship	84	33.9
Never had sexual intercourse	66	26.6
Number of sexual partners in past year		
0	70	28.2
1	92	37.1
2	35	14.1
3	21	8.5
4	12	4.8
5 or more	15	6.0
Condom use		
Always (100%)	85	34.3
Usually (76%–99%)	55	22.2
Sometimes (51%–75%)	20	8.1
Occasionally (26%–50%)	8	3.2
Rarely (1%–25%)	20	8.1
Never (0%)	34	13.7
Not answered	26	10.5
Oral contraceptive use		
Yes	136	54.8
No	109	44.0
Smoke cigarettes		
Yes	18	7.3
No	228	91.9
Last Papanicolaou test		
Never	72	29.0
Within the past year	154	62.1
Have not had in past year	21	8.5
PMH or FMH of HPV or cervical cancer		
Yes	52	21.0
No	193	77.8

Abbreviations: FMH, family medical history; PMH, past medical history.

or changes. More than 96% of these study participants identified multiple sex partners as a risk factor for cervical cancer. The primary areas of knowledge deficits identified in this population were risk factors for HPV (other than sexual intercourse) and signs and symptoms of HPV.

In these college sorority members there was no significant difference in knowledge regarding HPV and cervical cancer based on age ($F = 1.424$, $P = .227$). ANOVA was used to determine if there were mean differences in knowledge scores among the women currently in a sexual relationship; those who were previously sexually active, but not currently in a sexual relationship; and those who had never had sexual intercourse. There were no differences in knowledge among these groups ($F = 0.602$, $P = .548$). Knowledge scores were also examined for women who had never had a Pap; those who had a Pap in the past year; and those who had a Pap, but not in the past year. These mean differences did not reach significance at the $P = .05$ level ($F = 2.546$, $P = .080$).

No relationships were found in this group between HPV/cervical cancer knowledge and the number of sexual partners within the last year ($r = -0.072$, $P = .261$). Frequency of condom use also did not have any correlation with HPV and cervical cancer knowledge scores ($r = -0.029$, $P = .670$).

Finally, independent t-tests compared knowledge scores between different groups. No significant difference in HPV/cervical cancer knowledge was found between those who currently used oral contraceptives and those who did not ($F = 0.385$, $P = .536$), between those who currently smoked cigarettes and those who did not ($F = 0.732$, $P = .393$), or between those who had a personal or family history of diagnosis with HPV or cervical cancer and those who did not ($F = 0.370$, $P = .543$).

DISCUSSION

Female college sorority members in this study demonstrated high-risk sexual behaviors, with 33.4% having had 2 or more sexual partners in the past year. This rate is higher than that for female college students reported in the 2012 ACHA survey (22.1%). Condom use seemed to be more prevalent in this sample of sorority women than in the ACHA survey, with 56.5% reporting condom use usually or always; however, in this study women were asked a general question about condom use and not specifically about condom use with vaginal, anal, or oral sex.[8]

This sample of sorority members had relatively low knowledge levels regarding HPV and cervical cancer. However, this group showed more knowledge regarding HPV and cervical cancer than many other college students previously researched. The mean knowledge score for the sorority members was 10.7. Research by Ingledue and colleagues[28] used the same instrument and surveyed 428 college females. These investigators found an average knowledge score of only 6.8. When Denny-Smith and colleagues[27] used the same instrument and researched 240 female nursing students, the reported mean knowledge score for this group was 10.2. These findings support previous research findings of overall poor knowledge levels in college females regarding HPV, but indicate that the knowledge of these sorority members still surpassed other groups of their peers studied previously.

None of the variables tested in the present study were found to have any relationship with knowledge scores in this group of sorority members. The variables evaluated were age, sexual relationship status, number of sexual partners, use of condoms, use of oral contraceptives, use of cigarettes, frequency of Pap tests, and personal or family history of HPV or cervical cancer diagnosis. More research is needed in sorority females to find what factors may influence the HPV/cervical cancer knowledge levels of this group. Research with a larger sample may also be more likely to yield statistically significant results. The results of this study supported previous similar research in college females indicating overall poor knowledge levels regarding HPV and cervical cancer and high sexual risk behaviors. These research findings are particularly alarming because the highest prevalence of genital HPV infection is in college-age women. Low knowledge levels and risky sexual behaviors make college sorority members a group at high risk for HPV and other STDs. These results support a need for increased promotion of healthy sexual behaviors and STD prevention strategies for college sorority women. Increased knowledge of HPV and cervical cancer, increased uptake of HPV vaccination, and fewer sexually risky behaviors in college females could ultimately lead to fewer HPV infections and less cervical cancer.

Limitations

The relatively small sample size and convenience sampling method are limitations of this research. In addition, this research studied a very specific aggregate on college campuses (sorority females) at only one southern university and had a low response rate (9.74%). The survey did not ask questions regarding HPV vaccine status or intent to receive HPV vaccination. Social desirability response bias is a potential limitation, owing to the use of a self-report survey.

Implications for Future Research

Further research is essential in female college students and college-age females regarding sexual risk behaviors and knowledge of HPV/cervical cancer. Larger sample sizes, random sampling, sampling across universities, and sampling in different geographic regions could aid in adding to the body of knowledge on these topics. Further information about college females' knowledge and knowledge gaps regarding HPV, cervical cancer, and HPV vaccination could help to formulate effective intervention strategies that could increase HPV/cervical cancer knowledge and promote HPV vaccination. Randomized controlled trials using educational interventions must be completed to evaluate the best ways to increase HPV/cervical cancer knowledge and HPV vaccination rates in college females.

Implications for Clinical Practice

Prevention strategies at the primary and secondary level are essential in order to decrease the prevalence of HPV and to prevent cervical cancer. These health-promotion strategies need to include education, vaccination, and screening for cervical cancer. Vaccination for HPV following the ACIP recommendations has been established as the most effective primary HPV prevention strategy,[31] and the Pap smear remains the most effective screening method for cervical cancer in females. New recommendations for cervical cancer screening were released in March 2012 by both the US Preventive Services Task Force[32] and a multidisciplinary partnership among the American Cancer Society/American Society for Colposcopy and Cervical Pathology/American Society for Clinical Pathology.[33] Both groups concur that women younger than 21 years should not be screened for cervical cancer regardless of the age of sexual initiation or other risk factors, and that women aged 21 to 29 years should be screened with cytology alone every 3 years.[32,33]

Because HPV is contracted via sexual contact, HPV in men is also a significant epidemiologic problem even though the rates of morbidity and mortality related to HPV are lower in men than in women. The prevalence rate of HPV among heterosexual men is estimated at 20%, whereas rates for men who have sex with men can range from 2.9% to 12.7% depending on the area of the United States surveyed.[12] In October 2009, the quadrivalent HPV vaccine was approved for use in males aged 9 to 26 years,[34] and in the fall of 2011 the ACIP recommended that boys receive HPV vaccination at age 11 to 12. Young men 13 to 26 years old should begin the HPV series to catch up on the vaccinations.[34] There are no reported rates of HPV vaccination in boys and young men because the recommendation to vaccinate males was made only recently.[19]

Lack of knowledge about risks associated with sexual behavior and the cause of cervical cancer have been shown to be barriers to HPV vaccination and Pap-smear screening.[35-40] Therefore, education regarding HPV, HPV vaccination, cervical cancer, safe sexual practices (including condom use), and Pap-smear screening must be implemented. HPV and cervical cancer educational interventions are needed, with a focus on young men and women aged 12 to 26 years and on the parents of adolescents.[41,42] Worldwide, knowledge of HPV is generally poor.[41] This lack of knowledge about the prevalence, transmission, and sequelae of HPV is concerning because it may affect future health behaviors. Parent recommendation, health care provider recommendation, and knowledge of the consequences of HPV have all been shown to increase the uptake of HPV vaccination.[40] HPV education in video, written, text-message, and e-mail formats has been shown to increase HPV knowledge and vaccination intentions in young adults.[42,43]

Barriers to receiving recommended vaccines for both adolescent males and females include the need for preventive care visits, which are often not scheduled for this age group. There is also a need for additional visits to complete the recommended 3-shot series for the HPV vaccine. It is often difficult for primary care practices to identify and track the adolescents to assure compliance with the recommended vaccine schedule.[44] Stokely and colleagues[45] reported immunization rates based on 2009 National Immunization Survey-Teen, and noted that providers are not administering all of the recommended vaccinations at a vaccination visit. Among young girls aged 11 to 12 years who presented for vaccination visits, 64% did not receive the HPV vaccine.

Szilagyi and colleagues[44] conducted a randomized controlled trial with a multi-pronged approach, including a tiered tracking system, reminder/recall, and an outreach program, specifically targeted to the adolescent population. Through the use of these various interventions, they were able to demonstrate a 12% to 16% increased vaccination rate.[44]

The CDC has developed multiple products to help improve vaccination rates in teens. The CDC Web site includes information for parents, preteens and teens, health professionals, and public health professionals. This information includes multimedia products, references, publications, posters, flyers, information sheets, videos, health-tracking cards and Web features. Thirty-second video clips remind teens that they also need vaccinations. Health-e-Cards, a reminder system, have been developed for providers,

---

Box 2
What can YOU do to ensure your patients get fully vaccinated?

- Strongly recommend adolescent vaccines to parents of your 11- through 18-year-old patients. Parents trust your opinion more than anyone else's when it comes to immunizations. Studies consistently show that provider recommendation is the strongest predictor of vaccination.

- Use every opportunity to vaccinate your adolescent patients. Ask about vaccination status when they come in for sick visits and sports physicals.

- Patient reminder and recall systems such as automated postcards, phone calls, and text messages are effective tools for increasing office visits.

- Educate parents about the diseases that can be prevented by adolescent vaccines. Parents may know very little about pertussis, meningococcal disease, or HPV.

- Implement standing-order policies so that patients can receive vaccines without a health care provider examination or individual health care provider order.

From U.S. Department of Health and Human Services Centers for Disease Control and Prevention. Information for health care professionals about adolescent vaccines. Atlanta, GA: CDC; 2012. Available at: http://www.cdc.gov/vaccines/who/teens/downloads/hcp-factsheet.pdf. Accessed August 27, 2012.

parents, teens, and preteens. This information is also available in several languages including Spanish, Vietnamese, American Indian/Alaska Native, and Korean.[46]

SUMMARY

Health care providers and health educators need to grasp the significant scope of the problem of HPV in adolescents and young men and women, and implement strategies to improve HPV vaccination rates in individuals aged 26 years and younger (**Box 2**). Population-specific intervention strategies should be used in an effort to positively affect the sexual health of those at risk for HPV and its sequelae, and to promote sexually healthy lifestyles in the future. Health care providers must not only educate clients regarding HPV and cervical cancer but must also actively recommend vaccination as the most effective prevention strategy for HPV and cervical cancer.[39]

REFERENCES

1. Weinstock H, Berman S, Cates W Jr. Sexually transmitted diseases among American youth: incidence and prevalence estimates, 2000. Perspect Sex Reprod Health 2004;36(1):6–10.
2. Wong LP, Sam IC. Ethnically diverse female university students' knowledge and attitudes toward human papillomavirus (HPV), HPV vaccination and cervical cancer. Eur J Obstet Gynecol Reprod Biol 2010;148(1):90–5.
3. Hariri S, Unger E, Sternberg M, et al. Prevalence of genital human papillomavirus among females in the United States, the National Health and Nutrition Examination Survey, 2003-2006. J Infect Dis 2011;204(15):566–73.
4. Bosch FX, Burchell AN, Schiffman M, et al. Epidemiology and natural history of human papillomavirus infections and type-specific implications in cervical neoplasia. Vaccine 2008;26(Suppl 10):K1–16.
5. Datta SD, Koutsky LA, Ratelle S, et al. Human papillomavirus infection and cervical cytology in women screened for cervical cancer in the United States, 2003-2005. Ann Intern Med 2008;148(7):493–500.
6. Smith JS, Melendy A, Rana RK, et al. Age-specific prevalence of infection with human papillomavirus in females: a global review. J Adolesc Health 2008;43(4): S5–25.
7. Dunne EF, Unger ER, Sternberg M, et al. Prevalence of HPV infection among females in the United States. JAMA 2007;297(8):813–9.
8. American College Health Association. American College Health Association-National College Health Assessment II: Reference Group Executive Summary fall 2011. Hanover (MD): American College Health Association; 2012.
9. Steben M, Duarte-Franco E. Human papillomavirus infection: epidemiology and pathophysiology. Gynecol Oncol 2007;107(2 Suppl 1):S2–5.
10. Monk BJ, Tewari KS. The spectrum and clinical sequelae of human papillomavirus infection. Gynecol Oncol 2007;107(2 Suppl 1):S6–13.
11. Walboomers JM, Jacobs MV, Manos MM, et al. Human papillomavirus is a necessary cause of invasive cervical cancer worldwide. J Pathol 1999;189(1):12–9.
12. CDC. Epidemiology and prevention of vaccine-preventable diseases. The pink book. 12th edition. Atlanta (GA): CDC; 2012. Available at: http://www.cdc.gov/vaccines/pubs/pinkbook/hpv.html. Accessed August 14, 2012.
13. Stone KM, Karem KL, Sternberg MR, et al. Seroprevalence of human papillomavirus type 16 infection in the United States. J Infect Dis 2002;186(10):1396–402.
14. Snijders PJ, Steenbergen RD, Heideman DA, et al. HPV-mediated cervical carcinogenesis: concepts and clinical implications. J Pathol 2006;208(2):152–64.

15. Surveillance, Epidemiology, and End Results (SEER) Program. Prevalence database: "US estimated complete prevalence counts on 1/1/2004": National Cancer Institute DCCPS Surveillance Research Program Statistical Research and Applications Branch. 2007. Available at: http://seer.cancer.gov/cgi-bin/csr/1975_2009_pops09/search.pl. Accessed August 14, 2012.

16. WHO. Global burden of disease estimates for 2002. World Health Organization; 2002. Available at: http://www.who.int/healthinfo/global_burden_disease/estimates_regional_2002/en/index.html. Accessed August 14, 2012.

17. International Agency for Research on Cancer. Globocan 2002 database. International Agency for Research on Cancer; 2002. Available at: http://globocan.iarc.fr/. Accessed August 14, 2012.

18. American Cancer Society. What are the key statistics for cervical cancer? Updated 2004. Available at: http://www.cancer.org/cancer/cervicalcancer/index. Accessed August 14, 2012.

19. CDC. National survey shows HPV vaccine rates trail other teen vaccines. 2011. Available at: http://www.cdc.gov/media/releases/2011/p0825_hpv_vaccine.html. Accessed August 14, 2012.

20. Lucas JW, Schiller JS, Benson V. Summary health statistics for U.S. adults: National Health Interview Survey, 2001. Vital Health Stat 10 2004;(218):1–134.

21. United States Preventive Services Task Force (USPSTF). Guide to clinical preventive services: recommendations of the U.S. Preventive Services Task Force. Rockville (MD): Agency for Healthcare Research and Quality; 2009.

22. Dempsey AF, Gebremariam A, Koutsky LA, et al. Using risk factors to predict human papillomavirus infection: implications for targeted vaccination strategies in young adult women. Vaccine 2008;26(8):1111–7.

23. Viscidi RP, Kotloff KL, Clayman B, et al. Prevalence of antibodies to human papillomavirus (HPV) type 16 virus-like particles in relation to cervical HPV infection among college women. Clin Diagn Lab Immunol 1997;4(2):122–6.

24. Benning BR, Lund MR. Patient knowledge about human papillomavirus and relationship to history of abnormal Papanicolaou test results. J Low Genit Tract Dis 2007;11(1):29–34.

25. Yacobi E, Tennant C, Ferrante J, et al. University students' knowledge and awareness of HPV. Prev Med 1999;28(6):535–41.

26. D'Urso J, Thompson-Robinson M, Chandler S. HPV knowledge and behaviors of black college students at a historically black university. J Am Coll Health 2007; 56(2):159–63.

27. Denny-Smith T, Bairan A, Page MC. A survey of female nursing students' knowledge, health beliefs, perceptions of risk, and risk behaviors regarding human papillomavirus and cervical cancer. J Am Acad Nurse Pract 2006; 18(2):62–9.

28. Ingledue K, Cottrell R, Bernard A. College women's knowledge, perceptions, and preventive behaviors regarding human papillomavirus infection and cervical cancer. Am J Health Stud 2004;19(1):28–34.

29. Eberhardt D, Rice ND, Smith LD. Effects of Greek membership on academic integrity, alcohol abuse, and risky sexual behavior at a small college. NASPA Journal 2003;41(1):137–48.

30. Asel AM, Seifert TA, Pascarella ET. The effects of fraternity/sorority membership on college experiences and outcomes: a portrait of complexity. Oracle 2009;4(2).

31. Monsonego J, Cortes J, Greppe C, et al. Benefits of vaccinating young adult women with a prophylactic quadrivalent human papillomavirus (types 6, 11, 16 and 18) vaccine. Vaccine 2010;28:8065–72.

32. Moyer VA. Screening for cervical cancer: U.S. Preventive Services Task Force recommendation statement. Ann Intern Med 2012;156(12):880–91.
33. Saslow D, Solomon D, Lawson, HW, et al. The American Cancer Society, American Society for Colposcopy and Cervical pathology, and American Society for Clinical Pathology screening guidelines for the prevention and early detection of cervical cancer. CA: A Cancer Journal for Clinicians 2012;62(3):147–72.
34. CDC. 2010 Sexually transmitted diseases surveillance: other sexually transmitted diseases. 2011. Available at: http://www.cdc.gov/std/stats10/other.htm. Accessed August 14, 2012.
35. Klein P, Melinand C. Survey of mothers on human papillomavirus and diseases caused in 16 European countries: need for educational programmes. Paper presented at: 26th Annual Meeting of the European Society for Paediatric Infectious Diseases (ESPID). Graz (Austria), May 13–17, 2008.
36. Bynum SA, Brandt HM, Sharpe PA, et al. Working to close the gap: identifying predictors of HPV vaccine uptake among young African American women. J Health Care Poor Underserved 2011;22(2):549–61.
37. Blumenthal J, Frey MK, Worley MJ, et al. Adolescent understanding and acceptance of the HPV vaccination in an underserved population in New York City. J Oncol 2012;2012:904034.
38. Allen JD, Mohllajee AP, Shelton RC, et al. Stage of adoption of the human papillomavirus vaccine among college women. Prev Med 2009;48:420–5.
39. Bednarczyk RA, Birkhead GS, Morse DL, et al. Human papillomavirus vaccine uptake and barriers: association with perceived risk, actual risk and race/ethnicity among female students at a New York State university, 2010. Vaccine 2011;29:3138–43.
40. Bendik MK, Mayo RM, Parker VG. Knowledge, perceptions, and motivations related to HPV vaccination among college women. J Cancer Educ 2011;26:459–64.
41. Hilton S, Smith E. "I thought cancer was one of those random things. I didn't know cancer could be caught…": adolescent girls' understandings and experiences of the HPV programme in the UK. Vaccine 2011;29:4409–15.
42. Allen JD, Fantasia HC, Fontenot H, et al. College men's knowledge, attitudes, and beliefs about the human papillomavirus infection and vaccine. J Adolesc Health 2009;45:535–7.
43. Krawczyk A, Lau E, Perez S, et al. How to inform: comparing written and video education interventions to increase human papillomavirus knowledge and vaccination intentions in young adults. J Am Coll Health 2012;60(4):316–22.
44. Szilagyi PG, Humiston SG, Gallivan S, et al. Effectiveness of a citywide patient immunization navigator program on improving adolescent immunizations and preventive care visit rates. Arch Pediatr Adolesc Med 2011;165(6):547–53.
45. Stokely S, Cohn A, Jain N, et al. Compliance with recommendations and opportunities for vaccination at ages 11 to 12 years. Arch Pediatr Adolesc Med 2011;165(9):813–8.
46. CDC. Preteens and teens still need vaccines. 2011. Available at: http://www.cdc.gov/vaccines/who/teens/index.html. Accessed August 27, 2012.

Psychosocial Effects of Disaster in Children and Adolescents
Significance and Management

Sara L. Jones, PhD, RN, Cheryl K. Schmidt, PhD, RN, CNE, ANEF*

KEYWORDS

- Disaster preparedness • American Red Cross
- National Commission on Children and Disasters • Psychosocial effects
- Posttraumatic stress disorder in children

KEY POINTS

- Approximately 42% of children and adolescents are still in need of mental health services after disasters.
- Children respond to disaster in 3 distinct stages, with multiple factors affecting their vulnerability and resiliency.
- The primary concern is the symptom manifestation and development of posttraumatic stress disorder.
- The *National Commission on Children and Disasters 2010 Report* is an excellent resource for developing preparedness in all settings that provide care for youth.

INTRODUCTION

Societies throughout time have experienced their share of disasters, including community crises, natural disasters, and man-made catastrophes. Defined as a "calamitous event that generally involves injury or loss of life and destruction of property, generally outside the scope of normal human experiences, disasters occur on both small and large scales, affecting all populations."[1] In the last decade, the effects of such occurrences have been highlighted in the public eye. Events such as the terrorist attacks of 9/11 and Hurricane Katrina in the United States predominantly come to mind. The media publicized the massive physical and economic destruction, as well as the lives that were lost, which were apparent during these events, as

Disclosures: None.
College of Nursing, University of Arkansas for Medical Sciences, 4301 West Markham Street, #529, Little Rock, AR 72205, USA
* Corresponding author.
E-mail address: schmidtcherylk@uams.edu

individuals and communities joined in the rehabilitation efforts to aid the affected areas. Health care providers, trained volunteers, and average citizens emerged to again prove why we can still have faith in humanity. Although there is no denying the travesty of the events at the moment they occur and the immediate time thereafter, it is important to be aware of the long-term effects on the individuals involved.

Specifically, there are millions of children worldwide who have been exposed to such disasters. Some have been directly involved, whereas others have indirectly experienced the events through their families, communities, and the media. Current research has begun to explore the physical, psychological, and social effects on children and adolescents, finding many factors that affect the vulnerability and resiliency of this population. From firework explosions, brush fires, school shootings, city bombings, and terrorist attacks, to floods, hurricanes, tsunamis, and earthquakes, these traumatic events affect the lives of children and adolescents in multiple ways. This article provides a synthesis of the literature to address the psychosocial symptoms that present in children and adolescents after disasters, the factors that contribute to protecting children from these symptoms, and the implications for health care professionals to reduce the possibility of long-term psychopathologies.

BACKGROUND AND SIGNIFICANCE

In the last quarter century, the effects of many disasters on children and adolescents, including natural, technological, and man-made disasters that affect local, state, national, and international levels, have been discussed in the literature. Researchers have assessed these effects on youth at many different intervals of time, ranging from 3 months to 10 years after a disaster.[2,3] Assessment tools that have been used include (**Table 1**) the Post-Traumatic Stress Disorder Reaction Index (PTSD-RI), which is available in a children's version[4,5]; both of which are available in children's versions; the Hurricane-Related Traumatic Experience Questionnaire (HURTE)[4] and Earthquake Experience Questionnaire[6]; the Traumatic Exposure Severity Scale (TESS)[6,7] and Traumatic Stress Symptom Checklist[7]; the Children's Revised Impact of Event Scale (CRIES)[8,9]; and the Life Events Checklist.[4] and Depression Self-Rating Scale.[5] With approximately 42% of youth still in need of mental health services after a disaster, early assessments are necessary in order to identify the high-risk factors that may develop into psychological disorders.[1,10]

Children of different ages and developmental stages are affected differently by disaster. Although 1 study has found that symptoms of posttraumatic stress disorder (PTSD) were not influenced by age or grade in school,[7] another has found grade level to be the number 1 predictor of risk of PTSD.[11] In a study of 7832 children, grades 4 to 12, 6 months after 9/11, fourth-graders had significantly higher rates of PTSD symptom, as much as twice as many as fifth-graders.[11] Other literature supports this difference, although not to this extreme.

Although infants and toddlers are believed to be too young to cognitively comprehend a disaster, their family's response can disrupt their routine, causing regression and detachment.[12] Symptoms in toddlers commonly present in sleep disturbances, including night terrors and nightmares.[13] Behavior changes are apparent, and include clinginess and temper tantrums.[14] School-aged children's typical reactions are dominated by mood, anxiety, and behavioral changes. They are less able to understand the difference between an intentional act versus an unintentional incident and, hence, are more concerned with the consequences thereafter.[1] They tend to focus on the detail of the event and fear that more harm will occur. They rely heavily on their parents and primary caregiver to ensure safety. Adolescents, on the other hand, are more aware of

Table 1 Assessment tools		
Assessment Tool	**Acronym**	**Description of Tool**
Post-Traumatic Stress Disorder Reaction Index	PTSD-RI	Assesses PTSD symptoms per *Diagnostic and Statistical Manual of Mental Disorders* criteria
Children Post-Traumatic Disorder	CPTSD	Modifiable to include wording specific to traumatic event
Traumatic Exposure Severity Scales	TESS	Includes 2 sections: The occurrence of a range of traumatic experiences The amount of distress generated by each experience
Traumatic Stress Symptom Checklist	TSSC	Assesses for traumatic stress and depression symptoms Includes additional items to assess for distress and global disability
Children's Revised Impact of Event Scale	CRIES	Includes 3 sub-scales: Intrusion Avoidance Arousal
Hurricane-related Traumatic Experience Questionnaire	HURTE	Measures: Number of hurricane exposure experiences Amount of loss and disruption experienced immediately after the hurricane Continued loss and disruption long after hurricane
Earthquake Experience Questionnaire	EEQ	Includes 3 sections: Demographics, past traumas, psychiatric history, reason for being in vicinity of earthquake, and frequency of area after earthquake Location during earthquake, rubble experience, loss of family members, injury, level of fear, and experiences of other distress Resource loss, change in social support, and quality of social interactions
Other assessments include:		
Life Events Checklist (LEC)		Depression Self-Rating Scale
Posttraumatic Cognitions Inventory Test		Social Support Rating Scale

the logic behind intent and gravity of a natural catastrophe and are able to reason the implications of the event. Because of their past experiences, their behaviors can be more complicated and they may develop more anxiety and unrealistic fears. Although their parents are important, they rely more on friends and teachers for support. Helping others and contributing to the relief efforts help them cope.[7]

Stages of Children's Response to Disaster

When conducting assessments with youth, it is important to understand the normal recovery process after a disaster. Children have been found to respond in 3 distinct stages (**Table 2**). It is when symptoms persist into the third stage that mental health services are recommended. A child's first reaction immediately after a disaster consists of fright, disbelief, denial, and grief.[1] Many liken this response to the bereavement process.[15] Children also experience a sense of relief if loved ones survive. At this stage, if they believe that they are helping family members and others during the aftermath, they build resiliency. Resiliency refers to "good outcomes in spite of serious threats to adaptation or development."[16] Research focused on disasters identifies multiple factors that contribute to a child's ability to be resilient throughout the recovery process, with the number 1 factor being a strong social support system.[2,7,8] Protective factors that lead to resiliency and promotive factors that contribute to vulnerability are discussed later in this article.

A few days to several weeks after the disaster, stage 2 occurs, in which developmental regression may be manifested.[1] Many children show emotional distress, such as fear, anxiety, sadness, and isolation. Hyperactivity, aggression, and hostility toward others are also frequent. Studies have shown that it is more commonly girls who experience fear, anxiety, sadness, and isolation, are more expressive about their emotions, and have more frequent thoughts about the disaster, whereas boys show hyperactivity, aggression, and hostility toward others, have continued conduct problems, and require a longer period for recovery.[8,17,18] Sleep disturbances are also common at this stage. In a study of 5687 children and adolescents (ages 9–19 years), 35% reported sleep difficulties and 9% reported regularly occurring nightmares after Hurricane Hugo.[19] If sleep disturbances continue, there is an increased risk of developing disorders such as PTSD.

Table 2		
Youth stages of response to disaster or traumatic event		
	Stage	**Behaviors**
Stage 1	Immediately after disaster or traumatic event	Similar to the bereavement process Reactions of fright, disbelief, denial, and grief Sense of relief if loved ones are unharmed Crucial time for development of resiliency Resiliency built if able to help others
Stage 2	A few days to several weeks after the disaster or traumatic event	Developmental regression Sleep disturbances Hopelessness from future Emotional stress, including fear, anxiety, sadness, and isolation (more common in girls) Hyperactivity, aggression, and hostility (more common in boys)
Stage 3	Longer than 1 month after disaster or traumatic event	Behaviors have persistently continued without deescalation Accompanied by marked distress or behavior disorganization Symptoms that indicate development of PTSD Mental health services should be sought

Data from Hagan JF Jr. American Academy of Pediatrics Committee on Psychosocial Aspects of Child and Family Health, Task Force on Terrorism. Psychosocial implications of disaster or terrorism on children: a guide for the pediatrician. Pediatrics 2005;116(3):791.

Also during this second stage, children tend to show hopelessness toward the future, as reported in a study after a drought in a rural area of New South Wales.[20] After what was called the worst drought of the century, school-age children reported their perspectives of the event. Five of 7 of their top concerns were their families' health, familial relationships, their family farms not surviving financially, businesses and services being closed in their communities, and what their futures would hold if their family farms were lost, so much so that they considered leaving school to return home to help on the farm.

In the normal response process, these symptoms should start to decrease after 1 month. Stage 3 occurs when these responses continue longer and are accompanied by marked distress or behavior disorganization for longer than the first month after the disaster. At this time, mental health services should be sought.[1] The primary concern is the development of PTSD. Twenty-four and 30 months after Hurricane Katrina, 46% and 50% of youth ages 8 to 15 years reported sleep disturbances, and 25% and 16% reported fear of sleeping alone; of the total sample, 40% and 38% reported moderate to severe symptoms of PTSD.[13] PTSD is a disorder that follows exposure to an acute or chronic stressor that involves actual or threatened death or injury to an individual.[21] Immediate reactions are those of intense fear, disorganized or agitated behavior, or helplessness. Symptoms that follow include 3 distinct criteria that persist for at least 1 month: (1) persistent reexperience of the trauma, (2) avoidance of stimuli associated with the trauma and diminished general responsiveness, and (3) increased arousal or hypervigilance (**Box 1**). Manifestation of symptoms in children include loss of interest in pleasurable activities, irritability, loss of focus, hyperarousal, anxiety, nightmares, academic failure, delinquency, substance abuse, aggression, self-harm, withdrawal, and other somatic complaints.

The occurrence, severity, and duration of PTSD symptoms are apparent throughout the literature, although the prevalence rates vary between studies, ranging from 2.5%

Box 1
Diagnostic and Statistical Manual of Mental Disorders, Fourth Edition **diagnostic criteria for PTSD**

Exposure to a traumatic event in which both of the following were present:

- The person experienced an event that involved actual or threatened death or serious injury to themselves or others

- The person's response involved intense fear, helplessness, or horror

Disturbances cause clinically significant distress or impairment of at least 1-month duration

Symptoms include:

- Persistent reexperiencing of the traumatic event, including recollections, dreams, or a sense of reliving the event

- Persistent avoidance of stimuli associated with the trauma and numbing general responsiveness

- Persistent symptoms of increased arousal and hypervigilance, as indicated by difficulty with sleep, irritability or outbursts of anger, difficulty concentrating, or exaggerated startle response

Adapted from The American Psychiatric Association. Diagnostic and statistical manual of mental disorders. 4th edition, text revision. Washington, DC: The American Psychiatric Association; 2000; with permission.

to 90%.[9,19] For instance, 3 studies after earthquakes provide varying results. Ma and colleagues[9] evaluated the prevalence and predictor variables of PTSD 6 months after the Wenchuan earthquake in China in 2008.[9] In this study, 3208 adolescents (ages 12–18 years) were initially administered the CRIES test, along with a Posttraumatic Cognitions Inventory Test and Social Support Rating Scale. Three hundred and thirty-two who had CRIES scores greater than 30 (which indicates high rates of intrusion, avoidance, and hyperarousal) were then interviewed, of whom 79 (2.5%) of the total sample met the criteria for PTSD. Ayub and colleagues[8] found even higher rates of PTSD symptoms after the Kashmir earthquake of 2005 in Pakistan. Of 1154 children (ages 8–14 years), 64.8% had significant symptoms of PTSD, with girls more likely to manifest symptoms than boys.

In a longitudinal study after the Parnitha earthquake in Greece in 1999, adolescents (in junior and high school) were evaluated for PTSD, depression, and quality of life (QOL) after 3 months and then again after 32 months.[5,22] At 3 months, among 1937 children and adolescents, PTSD rates were estimated at 4.5% and clinical depression at 13.9%, with PTSD scores being the single most powerful variable predicting depression.[22] At 32 months, 511 adolescents from the initial study were assessed. Most PTSD symptoms were reported at mild levels, but 8.8% of the children and adolescents were still experiencing moderate to severe levels of PTSD and 13.6% met criteria for clinical depression.[5] PTSD symptoms at moderate to severe levels were most highly correlated with frequency of experiencing reminders of the earthquake in the past month (15%). Girls reported hearing sounds, seeing signs of destruction, and seeing faces that reminded them of the earthquake twice as much and more often than boys. Twenty-seven percent of girls and 11% of boys had experienced 2 or more reminders in the preceding month. Lower levels of QOL predicted greater levels of PTSD and depression.

Estimated rates of PTSD in youth varied after Hurricane Katrina as well. Some report as many as 50% with symptoms of emotional disturbances for up to 6 months after Katrina, but some suggest that these symptoms are short-lived after this time frame.[23,24] McLaughlin and colleagues[23] interviewed 797 children (ages 4–17 years) 27 months after the hurricane, finding 15% to be experiencing serious emotional disturbances, including aggression, self-injury, excessive fear, anxiety, withdrawal, learning difficulties, and PTSD.[23] After 36 to 39 months, 11% continued to have these experiences.

Moore and Varela[4] surveyed a smaller sample of 156 fourth-graders, fifth-graders, and sixth-graders 33 months after Hurricane Katrina. Forty-six percent self-reported moderate to very severe levels of PTSD symptoms. These symptoms were correlated with the child's experience of the hurricane, using the HURTE, which indicated the child's level of exposure to the hurricane (ie, saw house destroyed, witnessed someone getting hurt), level of immediate loss or disruption (ie, home damaged, had to move), and continued loss and disruption (ie, parent unemployed, multiple moves) after the hurricane. The number of negative life events was found to be directly related to PTSD symptoms.

Other studies include rates of PTSD in youth after a wildfire and a tsunami. Students (ages 7–12 years) were evaluated 6 months after a wildfire in Greece that killed a total of 67 people, destroyed 815 houses, and injured many people.[25] Probable PTSD symptoms were present in 29.4%, and another 20% had symptoms of probable depression. Four and a half years after a tsunami in Japan, 482 adolescent survivors (ages 11–19 years) were administered the CPTSD and TESS.[7] Long after this event, moderate to very severe symptoms of PTSD occurred in 63% of the participants. Again, girls showed more frequent and severe symptoms.

Protective and Promotive Factors

It is estimated that approximately 25% of adults who experience disasters develop PTSD, but the risk posed to children and adolescents can differ greatly because of their individual vulnerabilities and resiliencies.[1] Previous experiences of direct exposure or witnessing trauma can increase one's resiliency and ability to cope with adversity; it can also increase one's sensitivity to trauma, rendering a worse, more intense response.[16] Many promotive and protective factors have been identified that contribute to the risk of youth developing PTSD after a disaster.[16] Three months after Hurricane Andrew, Vernberg and colleagues[2] developed a conceptual model after examining the symptoms of 568 elementary school-aged children. These investigators identified 4 primary factors that accounted for 62% of their PTSD symptoms, including: exposure to traumatic events, child characteristics, access to social support, and children's coping. Specific negative life events related to exposure to a disaster that have been found to directly influence the severity of PTSD symptoms include witnessing destruction, changing schools, losing a home, and staying in a shelter.[4] Symptoms are more severe when the events are ongoing.

Gender is also identified as a moderator of risk versus resiliency. Females repeatedly report greater experiences of distress and more severe levels of PTSD after a disaster.[16] Also, there is a difference in the type of symptoms that present in males versus females. Whereas males more often have externalized symptoms, females report internalized symptoms. Eighteen months after the Kashmir earthquake in Pakistan, when 64.8% of children had significant symptoms of PTSD, 35% of girls and 25% of boys had emotional disorders, and 16.1% of boys and 10.1% of girls met criteria for hyperactivity.[8] Other characteristics that affect the vulnerability of children after living through a disaster include personality traits, such as preexisting anxiety, negative emotionality, or a shy nature, which increase vulnerability.[1]

Access to social support affects a child's response immediately after a disaster long thereafter, whether it comprises parents, family members, teachers, friends, or community.[2] Support systems are effective because of their ability to minimize negative beliefs and calm fears, along with enabling problem solving and encouraging positive behaviors.[7] Specifically, loss of a parent is one of the most significant factors that influence severity of PTSD symptoms; how parents respond to the disaster also affects the child's responses.[7] Studies show that parents play a significant role in a child's ability to adjust after a traumatic event.[26] Immediately after 9/11, rates of PTSD in adults doubled compared with other disasters, but within 3 months, rates declined in two-thirds of the population.[27] However, it was during those 3 months that children were most dependent on their parents for emotional and psychological needs, which the parents were less able to meet because of their own distress. Further, when both children and parents were questioned about the child's symptoms, the parent's level of PTSD symptoms correlated with their report of their child's symptoms.[12]

Children involved in therapy after these experiences often use themes from the events in their play.[28] Even 10 years after the attacks on the World Trade Center on 9/11, therapists continued to report the symbolic play, enactments, and drawings by children who not only directly witnessed the attacks but also saw them on television. Media exposure significantly contributes to a child's response to trauma. One study with 248 elementary school students evaluated the effects of media coverage of disastrous weather on levels of anxiety.[29] State anxiety was significantly higher in children shown disaster media cues compared with those shown neutral weather, even in the absence of direct disaster exposure. In these cases, levels of anxiety were significantly related to perceived social support and coping strategies.

CLINICAL IMPLICATIONS

A key strategy in helping children and adolescents cope with disasters is to involve them directly in preparedness activities. Many voluntary and official organizations have developed programs to accomplish this goal. See **Box 2** for the names and Web sites of the most successful programs. In the aftermath of September 11, 2001, the American Red Cross developed an entire curriculum called *Masters of Disaster* to help children in grades from kindergarten to high school to understand and prepare for a variety of disasters.[30] As children mature, they can explore the Internet independently to learn about disasters and develop plans specific to their schools and communities. For example, children may lead a collection drive for supplies to shelter in place in their schools if a disaster makes it impossible to leave or have replacement supplies delivered. A day care center needs to stockpile at least a few days' worth of food, water, diapers, and other essential supplies in case a disaster requires sheltering in place. If the disaster requires evacuation, are all children identified with an ankleband or wristband for eventual reunification with family? These simple steps go a long way toward preventing the psychological distress of

---

Box 2
Resources for preparing youth for disasters

Administration for Children and Families (2009) *Head Start Emergency Preparedness Manual.* US Department of Health and Human services. Washington, DC: HHS.

American Academy of Pediatrics, the American Public Health Association, and the National Resource Center for Health and Safety in Child Care (2005) *Emergency/Disaster Preparedness for Child Care Programs: Caring for Our Children–National Health and Safety Performance Standards: Guidelines for Out-of-Home Child Care Applicable Standards.* From http://nrc.uchsc. edu. Accessed October 18, 2012.

American Red Cross (2007) *Masters of Disaster Educator's Kit.* From http://www.shopstaywell. com/. Accessed October 18, 2012.

American Red Cross (2011) *The American Red Cross Ready Rating Program.* From http://www. redcross.org/. Accessed October 18, 2012.

Discovery Education (2011) *Ready Classroom.* From http://readyclassroom.discoveryeducation. com. Accessed October 18, 2012.

Federal Emergency Management Agency (2010) *Ready Kids.* From http://www.ready.gov/kids. Accessed October 18, 2012.

National Commission on Children and Disasters (2010, October) *2010 Report to the President and Congress.* AHRQ publication no. 10-MO37. Rockville, MD: Agency for Healthcare Research and Quality.

North American Mission Board, Southern Baptist Convention Disaster Relief, *Church Preparedness for Disaster,* available through Google online search.

O'Brien M, Webster S, Herrick A (2007) *Coping with Disasters and Strengthening Systems: A Framework for Child Welfare Agencies.* From http://muskie.usm.maine.edu/helpkids/rcpdfs/ coping with disasters.pdf. Accessed October 18, 2012.

Portune L, Gatowski SI (2008) *Ensuring the unique needs of dependency courts are met in disaster planning efforts: dependency court planning templates for continuity of operations plans.* (Reno, NV: National Council of Juvenile and Family Court Judges and American Bar Association). From http://www.ncjfcj.org/. Accessed October 18, 2012.

US Department of Education (2009) *Action Guide for Emergency Management at Institutions of higher education.* From http://rems.ed/gov/docs/REMS_Action Guide.pdf. Accessed October 18, 2012.

being separated from family. In the immediate aftermath of Hurricane Katrina, news clips filmed at the Superdome in New Orleans showed mothers passing their infants, wearing only diapers because of the heat and humidity, over the heads of others, saying "Save my child–I'll catch up later." It took several months for some of those mothers to be reunited with their children. Parents need advice on how to identify their children during mass evacuation events, even a simple technique such as putting the parent's name and phone number on the child's chest or back with a marker.

All facilities that house or serve children and adolescents for even a few hours a day are ethically obligated to make plans to protect them during and after disasters. The Agency for Healthcare Research and Quality established the National Commission on Children and Disasters, which published an Interim Report in 2009 and a Final Report in 2010 to the President and Congress.[31] These reports spelled out detailed recommendations and responsible agencies for ensuring the safety of children in schools and other congregate child care settings. Those recommendations include the 3 phases of preparedness, response, and recovery and provide extensive resources for personnel in a variety of settings to tap when developing plans for dealing with disasters.

Exploring the entire 2010 National Commission Report is beyond the scope of this article.[31] The report includes 11 recommendations, with several subrecommendations under each, covering the major categories of (1) disaster management and recovery, (2) mental health, (3) child physical health, (4) emergency medical services and pediatric transport, (5) disaster case management, (6) child care and early education, (7) elementary and secondary education, (8) child welfare and juvenile justice, (9) sheltering standards, services, and supplies, (10) housing, and (11) evacuation. Each of these recommendations includes detailed descriptions of how communities should meet the needs of children during disasters and which government agencies are responsible for insuring that these activities occur. For instance, recommendation 2.3 under "Mental health" states:

Federal agencies and nonfederal partners should enhance pre-disaster preparedness and just-in-time training in pediatric disaster mental health and behavioral health, including psychological first aid, bereavement support, and brief supportive interventions, for mental health professionals and individuals, such as teachers, who work with children.

If this recommendation had been in place before the disasters described earlier in this article, imagine the impact it might have had on the psychological reactions children and adolescents experienced.

The American Red Cross follows detailed policies and procedures to protect children in disaster shelters. For example, children stay with their parents or guardians at all times while in the shelter, unless the latter authorize an approved child care volunteer to supervise their children in a designated area of the shelter. If a child is separated from parents or guardians, the Red Cross shelter staff refer the child to the local Department of Human Services or Child Protective Services for care and follow-up. Age-appropriate games, art materials, and a television or DVD player are provided whenever possible. Red Cross Health Services and Disaster Mental Health Services staff and volunteers are available to assist children and adolescents in coping with the effects of the disaster. In long-term shelters, the Red Cross makes arrangements for children to be transported to their own or a local school. It is important to provide as much routine as possible for children and adolescents, to decrease their stress and help them regain a sense of normalcy.

SUMMARY

This article explores the potential short-term and long-term psychosocial conse-quences of disasters in children and adolescents and offers a variety of strategies to help them cope and recover from the effects of these disasters. More research is needed to determine the relative effectiveness of various strategies in helping children to prepare for, respond to, and recover from disasters. Nurses need to be actively involved in developing evidence-based protocols that can be implemented by fami-lies, communities, and public health and social agencies.

The primary theme in preparing and caring for children and adolescents in disas-ters should be prevention. If families, caretakers, teachers, and others who work with children and adolescents can anticipate the potential impact of disasters, it may be possible to delay or even prevent some of the negative consequences of disasters.

REFERENCES

1. Hagan J. Psychosocial implications of disaster or terrorism on children: a guide for the pediatrician. Pediatrics 2005;116:787–95.
2. Vernberg E, La Greca A, Silverman W, et al. Prediction of posttraumatic stress symptoms in children after Hurricane Andrew. J Abnorm Psychol 1996;105(2):237–48.
3. Pfefferbaum B, Tucker P, North C, et al. Physiological reactivity in children of Oklahoma City. Ann Clin Psychiatry 2011;23(3):202–7.
4. Moore K, Varela R. Correlates in long-term posttraumatic stress symptoms in chil-dren following Hurricane Katrina. Child Psychiatry Hum Dev 2010;41:239–50.
5. Goenijan A, Roussos A, Steinberg A, et al. Longitudinal study of PTSD, depres-sion, and quality of life among adolescents after the Parnitha earthquake. J Affect Disord 2011;122:509–15.
6. Kihc C, Zinnur Kihc E, Orhan Aydin I. Effects of relocation and parental psycho-pathology on earthquake survivor-children's mental health. J Nerv Ment Dis 2011;199(5):335–41.
7. Agustini EN, Asniar I, Matsuo H. The prevalence of long-term post-traumatic stress symptoms among adolescents after the tsunami in Aceh. J Psychiatr Ment Health Nurs 2011;18:543–9.
8. Ayub M, Poongan I, Masood K, et al. Psychological morbidity in children 18 months after Kashmir Earthquake of 2005. Child Psychiatry Hum Dev 2012;43:323–36.
9. Ma X, Liu X, Hu X, et al. Risk indicators for post-traumatic stress disorder in adolescents exposed to the 5.12 Wenchuan Earthquake in China. Psychiatry Res 2010;189:385–91.
10. Osofsky JD, Osofsky HJ, Harris WW. Katrina's children: social policy consider-ations for children in disasters. Soc Policy Rep 2007;21:3–18.
11. Rosen CS, Cohen M. Subgroups of New York City children at high risk of PTSD after the September 11 attacks: a signal detection analysis. Psychiatr Serv 2010;61:64–9.
12. Boer F, Smith C, Morren M, et al. Impact of a technological disaster on young chil-dren: a five-year postdisaster multi-informant study. J Trauma Stress 2009;22(6):516–24.
13. Brown T, Mellman T, Alfano C, et al. Sleep fears, sleep disturbance, and PTSD symptoms in minority youth exposed to Hurricane Katrina. J Trauma Stress 2011;24(5):575–80.

14. Veenema TG, Schroeder-Bruce K. The aftermath of violence: children, disaster, and posttraumatic stress disorder. J Pediatr Health Care 2002;16:235–44.
15. Schmidt CK, Terry D, Dorman D, et al. Disaster nursing in schools and other community congregate child care settings. In: Disaster nursing and emergency preparedness: for chemical, biological, and radiological terrorism and other hazards. 3rd edition. New York: Springer; 2013. p. 581–613.
16. Masten A, Narayan A. Child development in the context of disaster, war, and terrorism: pathways of risk and resilience. Annu Rev Psychol 2012;63:227–57.
17. Pine DS, Cohen JA. Trauma in children and adolescents: risk and treatment of psychiatric sequelae. Biol Psychiatry 2002;51:519–31.
18. American Academy of Pediatrics, Work group on disasters. Psychological issues for children and families in disasters: a guide for the primary care physician. Washington, DC: US Department of Health and Human Services; 1995.
19. Shannon MP, Lonigan CJ, Finch AJ Jr, et al. Children exposed to disaster: epidemiology of post-traumatic symptoms and symptom profiles. J Am Acad Child Adolesc Psychiatry 1994;33:80–93.
20. Carnie T, Berry H, Blinkhorn S, et al. In their own words: young people's mental health in drought affected rural and remote NSW. Aust J Rural Health 2011;19: 244–8.
21. American Psychiatric Association. Diagnostic and statistical manual of mental disorders. 4th edition, text revised. Washington, DC: American Psychiatric Association; 2000.
22. Roussos A, Goenjian A, Steinberg A, et al. Posttraumatic stress and depressive reactions among children and adolescents after the 1999 earthquake in Ano Liosia, Greece. Am J Psychiatry 2005;162:530–7.
23. McLaughlin KA, Fairbank JA, Gruber MJ, et al. Serious emotional disturbance among youth exposed to Hurricane Katrina 2 years postdisaster. J Am Acad Child Adolesc Psychiatry 2009;48(11):1069–78.
24. Murray JS. Children of Hurricane Katrina. Disaster care. Am J Nurs 2011;111(8): 52–5.
25. Papadatou D, Giannopoulou I, Bitsakou P, et al. Adolescents' reactions after a wildfire disaster in Greece. J Trauma Stress 2012;25:57–63.
26. Eisenberg N, Silver R. Growing up in the shadow of terrorism: youth in America after 9/11. Am Psychol 2012;66(6):468–81.
27. Galea S, Resnick H, Vlahov D. Psychological sequelae of September 11 [letter]. N Engl J Med 2002;347:444.
28. Aiello T. What the children said: children's narrative constructions of the events of 9/11 in psychotherapy. J Infant Child Adolesc Psychother 2011;11:32–8.
29. Ortiz C, Silverman W, Jaccard J, et al. Children's state anxiety in reaction to disaster media cures: a preliminary test of a multivariate model. Psychological Trauma: Theory, Research, Practice and, Policy 2011;3(2):157–64.
30. American Red Cross. Masters of disaster educator's kit. 2007. Available at: http://www.shopstaywell.com/. Accessed October 18, 2012.
31. National Commission on Children and Disasters. 2010 Report to the President and Congress. AHRQ publication no. 10-MO37. Rockville (MD): AHRQ Publication; 2010.

Challenges in Providing Preventive Care To Inner-City Children with Asthma

Arlene M. Butz, ScD, MSN[a,b,*], Joan Kub, PhD, MSN[b],
Melissa H. Bellin, PhD, LCSW[c], Kevin D. Frick, PhD[d]

KEYWORDS

- Asthma • Inner city • Preventive care

KEY POINTS

- Major challenges to preventive asthma care are encountered by inner-city children and include family and patient attitudes and beliefs, lack of access to quality medical care, and psychosocial and environmental factors.
- Pediatric nurses can affect these challenges by identifying parental attitudes and beliefs about asthma medications, parental depression and stress, and environmental exposures. Remediation of these challenges may require referral to community resources such as an asthma specialist, community mental health clinics, and smoking-cessation clinics.
- Alternative or supplemental health care sites such as school-based asthma programs, community or mobile health care clinics, or disease case management programs may enhance access to preventive care for high-risk inner-city children.

INTRODUCTION

Asthma affects 7.1 million children in the United States and is the number 1 cause of pediatric emergency department (ED) visits.[1–3] Although the scientific understanding of the pathophysiology of asthma and the quality of asthma therapies have significantly improved over the past 30 years, asthma morbidity remains high and preventive care low for inner-city children. Low-income, African American children have a 4.1-times higher rate of ED visits and a death rate 7.6 times higher than rates of non-Hispanic white children,[4] although minority low-income children are the least

[a] Department of Pediatrics, The Johns Hopkins University School of Medicine, 200 North Wolfe Street, Baltimore, MD 21287, USA; [b] Department of Community Health, School of Nursing, Johns Hopkins University, 525 North Wolfe street, Baltimore, MD 21287, USA; [c] School of Social Work, The University of Maryland at Baltimore, 525 West Redwood Street, Baltimore, MD 21201, USA; [d] Department of Health Policy and Management, The Johns Hopkins University Bloomberg School of Public Health, 615 North Wolfes Street, Baltimore, MD 21205, USA
* Corresponding author. Division of General Pediatrics, Johns Hopkins University School of Medicine, 200 North Wolfe Street Room 2051, Baltimore, MD 21287.
E-mail address: abutz@jhmi.edu

Nurs Clin N Am 48 (2013) 241–257
http://dx.doi.org/10.1016/j.cnur.2013.01.008
0029-6465/13/$ – see front matter © 2013 Elsevier Inc. All rights reserved.

likely to receive adequate guideline-based therapy.[5–7] Furthermore, Hispanic and black children have higher rates of inadequate health care insurance in comparison with white children.[8] This disparity in asthma morbidity among inner-city children often results from inadequacies of the health care delivery system[8] as well as from individual factors regarding the patient, caregiver, and health care provider.

Preventive asthma care among inner-city children is challenging because of a variety of factors including health care system/organizational and provider characteristics, patient and family attitudes and beliefs, and psychosocial and environmental factors. These factors affect a child's opportunity to receive preventive care for asthma and, if missed, can result in increased asthma morbidity and health care costs (**Fig. 1**). Specific health care system/organizational challenges are lack of access to quality medical care, including long wait times and unavailability of health care appointments, lack of transportation to clinic sites, and lack of access to specialty asthma care. Especially challenging to preventive care for inner-city children with asthma is nonadherence to national asthma guidelines by health care providers. Self-reported rates of adherence of primary care providers to national asthma guidelines are low,[9–11] and may lead to misclassification of asthma severity and control for the child owing to unfamiliarity with guidelines. This misclassification of severity may contribute to the underuse of anti-inflammatory medications consistently reported in inner-city children.[12–15] Family and patient attitudes and beliefs about asthma care, psychosocial factors including caregiver depression and life stress,[16–19] and environmental factors found in the child's home and neighborhood are other major challenges to preventive asthma care in inner-city children. This article purposely focuses on 4 major challenges to providing preventive care (family and patient attitudes and beliefs, lack of access to quality medical care, psychosocial factors, and environmental factors) based on prior evidence and the authors' own observation of these challenges in research with inner-city children with asthma over the past decade. Pediatric nurses are in contact with children with asthma and their families in a variety of settings including schools, community health, primary care, EDs, and inpatient units. The goal of this article is to describe the aforementioned challenges, address cost issues related to preventive care, and provide recommendations for pediatric nurses across settings.

CHALLENGES TO PREVENTIVE ASTHMA CARE
Caregiver/Family Attitudes and Beliefs About Asthma Care

Common caregiver/family attitudes and beliefs about asthma preventive care are (1) lack of appreciation for preventive asthma medication and follow-up care when a child with asthma is asymptomatic, and (2) distrust and worry about side effects of medications.[5,20,21] The evidence from several studies indicates that even when appropriate preventive asthma medications are prescribed, only 30% to 50% of children with asthma who require daily preventive medications receive adequate doses anti-inflammatory medications.[13,14,22] The most common contributor to nonadherence to daily preventive medication use in children with asthma is misunderstanding by both caregiver and child of the role of daily anti-inflammatory medications in treating asthma. For instance, caregivers may believe that the child's asthma is not severe enough to require daily medication, noted in many nonadherent adult patients with asthma[21] and consistent with caregiver reports of high symptom days but low use of daily preventive medications by their children.[6,14,23] Moreover, administration of daily preventive medications is complex, with complicated regimens and delivery systems. Accurate use of metered dose inhalers (MDIs), dry powder inhalers, and nebulizers requires cooperation and coordination from the child. The use of spacers

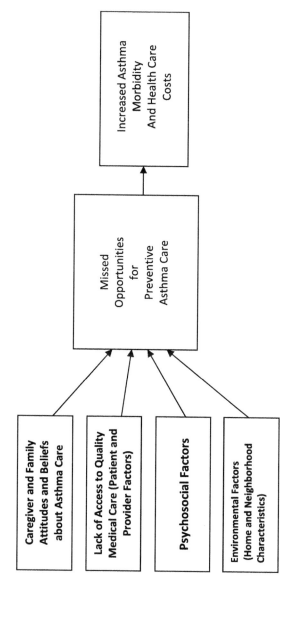

Fig. 1. Challenges to preventive care for inner-city children with asthma.

with MDIs significantly enhances aerosolized medication deposition into the lung instead of the mouth or pharynx, and is recommended for use by all children and adolescents who are prescribed MDI-administered asthma medications.

Parental worry about medication dependence and reduced effectiveness of long-term use of asthma medications has been reported.[14,21] In the authors' current study of 300 inner-city children aged 3 to 10 years with persistent asthma and frequent ED visits for asthma, nearly one-third of parents reported that they were very worried about the side effects of their child's asthma medications (**Table 1**). This level of parental worry is most likely related to concerns of potential long-term effects, misperception of the type of steroid medication (nonanabolic steroid), and the perceived risk of dependence.[25]

Child age appears to be associated with adherence to preventive care appointments because of the competing demands of school and work. In the authors' behavioral intervention study of children with persistent asthma, younger children were significantly more likely to attend a primary care follow-up visit for asthma than older children, most likely because competing school or work obligations of older children impeded attending an appointment with the primary care physician during daytime hours.[26] Alternatively, caregivers may be more concerned about asthma symptoms and acute exacerbations in younger children who are less able to communicate their asthma symptoms or unable to communicate their symptoms as clearly as older children. Furthermore, because older children may self-manage their asthma, parental awareness of symptoms may be decreased.

Guideline-based asthma treatment is based on accurate recognition and reporting of symptoms by the family, and appropriate classification of severity by the health care provider. A critical premise of effective asthma self-management is the caregiver's and/or child's ability to communicate the symptom level to the health care provider and have the provider accurately assign a severity level that indicates treatment guidelines. Communication about asthma severity may be impaired by poor symptom perception on the part of the child or parent,[27,28] or inappropriate symptom labeling by the parent or health care provider. For example, mislabeling cough as nonasthma may result in misdiagnosis and inadequate treatment of asthma. Perceptions of asthma symptoms by parents and children are multidimensional and include nonspecific symptoms such as fatigue, malaise, and fear.[29] Miscommunication about symptom frequency and severity between parents and providers may result in an inaccurate assessment of severity, leading to an inappropriate medication regimen and uncontrolled asthma.[13]

Recommendations to improve understanding of caregiver/family attitudes and beliefs about asthma care

- Identify and discuss parental attitudes, beliefs, and worries about medications, including potential side effects and dependence on asthma medications.
- Teach parents and school-age children specific and nonspecific symptoms of asthma, and identify descriptors of child symptoms for parents and teachers to use.
- Monitor younger and newly diagnosed children with asthma more frequently through the evolving ability of the parent and child to recognize asthma symptoms.[27,30]

Lack of Access to Quality Medical Care: Patient and Health Care Provider Factors

Common health care system/organizational barriers to preventive care encountered by inner-city children with asthma include lack of available primary care appointments, long wait times or inconvenient times for scheduled appointments,[31,32] lack of endorsement by the child's primary care provider for the need to follow up after ED visits,[33,34] lack of transportation, lack of affordable child care, fear of losing one's job through attending multiple medical appointments, and lack of referral to specialty care for treatment when indicated.[23]

Several behavioral interventions targeting system/organizational barriers have shown modest improvement in providing preventive asthma care; these include school-based screening, health care provider prompting for guideline-based care, and parent Web-based feedback interventions.[35–39] Successful physician feedback interventions for asthma include providing feedback on specific asthma health information to the child's primary care provider regarding the child's symptom frequency and frequency of ED visits,[15] and information sent by providers regarding their patients' adherence to inhaled corticosteroid (ICS) use as compared with prescribed doses.[38] Although case management, another successful organizational intervention for high-risk children, is usually reimbursable, it is not standard practice in all health care settings. Moreover, case management is often inadequately structured to have any significant impact on inner-city children with complex social problems such as family mental health issues[18] or poor-quality housing.

Alternative health care delivery models, such as school-based and mobile health vans, have shown potential in tackling system/organizational barriers to preventive care for inner-city children with asthma. One promising intervention is an asthma therapy program consisting of monitoring asthma control and administering daily preventive medications, which is delivered in public schools.[39] Based on the research team's prior successful model using directly observed therapy (DOT) of preventive medications to children with persistent asthma by school health staff,[39] the asthma therapy intervention was improved by the addition of a Web-based communication between an asthma care coordinator, the child's health care provider, and the school. The intervention is integrated within school and community systems, and pilot data indicate that the majority of children received preventive medications during school hours.[40]

Use of mobile health vans is increasing in popularity as a way to improve access to care for a variety of medical and dental diseases.[41,42] The mobile clinics are predominantly used at schools that offer the advantages of providing multiple sites for care, eliminating transportation issues and resulting in a decrease in missed appointments.[42] The Breathmobile program, a mobile health clinic providing specialty asthma care, is an innovative solution to help increase access to specialty care for underserved children with asthma.[43] Children attending the Baltimore Breathmobile had a significant reduction in symptom-free days, urgent care visits, and improved controller medication use, and has proved to be an effective model of health care delivery for underserved children.[41]

Nonadherence by health care providers to national asthma guidelines is another significant challenge to preventive care for inner-city children with asthma. More than a decade ago, national asthma guidelines were published by the National Heart, Lung, and Blood Institute (NHLBI) National Asthma Education and Prevention Program (NAEPP) in an attempt to standardize and improve the quality of asthma care and to disseminate best practices for asthma management.[44] However, provision of preventive asthma medication is strikingly low in minority inner-city children,[5] with rates of anti-inflammatory medication use of between 40% and 60% for inner-city children with persistent asthma.[9,45] Less than half (44%) receive a written asthma action plan, only half (51%) receive advice regarding environmental control,[7] and only 23% to 24% of these children are seen by an asthma specialist.[23,46] Despite most pediatricians (88%) indicating awareness and access to the guidelines, there is a wide gap

Table 1
Baseline characteristics of inner-city children with persistent asthma enrolled in pediatric asthma alert intervention (N = 300)

Characteristic	Number (%)
Child's age	
Mean (SD)	5.65 (2.2)
Race/Ethnicity	
African American	286 (95.4)
Hispanic/Latino	3 (1.0)
White	4 (1.3)
Other	7 (2.3)
Health insurance type	
Medicaid	275 (91.7)
Private	24 (8.0)
Self-pay	1 (0.3)
Caregiver Characteristics	
Caregiver age	
Mean (SD)	31.5 (7.0)
Marital status	
Single	210 (70.0)
Married	56 (18.7)
Other	34 (11.3)
Center for Epidemiologic Studies Depression Scale (n = 298)	
$\geq$16 (Clinical cutoff for depressive symptoms)	102 (34.2)
Caregiver Daily Life Stress	
Mean (SD) (Range: 0 = No stress and 10 = high stress)	6.33 (2.9)
Caregiver Asthma Life Stress	
Mean (SD) (Range: 0 = No stress and 10 = high stress)	5.16 (3.7)
Child Health Characteristics	
Symptom days past 2 wk	
0–3	98 (32.7)
4 or more (not controlled)	202 (67.3)
Symptom nights (n = 299)	
0–2	101 (33.8)
3 or more (not controlled)	198 (66.2)
Number of ED visits for asthma past 6 mo	
None	13 (4.4)
1–2	157 (52.3)
3 or more	130 (43.3)
Routine preventive asthma care visits past 6 mo	
None	29 (9.7)
1	75 (25.0)
2	76 (25.3)
3 or more	120 (40.0)
Seen by asthma specialist last 2 y	
Yes	58 (19.3)
Asthma Action Plan in the home	
Yes	103 (34.3)
Uses a spacer for inhaled medications	
Yes	276 (92.0)
Uses a peak flow meter in home	
Yes	73 (24.3)

(continued on next page)

Characteristic	Number (%)
Table 1 *(continued)*	
Uses home remedies for asthma (n = 296)	
Yes	100 (33.8)
Worried or concerned about child's asthma medications and side effects[a] (n = 299)	
Very, very worried or very worried	92 (30.8)
Fairly or somewhat or a little worried	65 (21.7)
Hardly or not worried	142 (47.5)
Smoker in the home	
Yes	177 (59.0)
Cockroaches in the home	
Yes	84 (28.0)
Mice in the home	
Yes	137 (45.7)
Violence exposure (seeing violence in the neighborhood)	69 (23.0)

[a] Item from Pediatric Asthma Caregivers Quality of Life Questionnaire.[24]

between preventive care of children with asthma and the NAEPP guidelines, with low rates of adherence by primary care providers.[9–11] Rates of 39% to 53% have been reported for specific guideline components: 53% for prescribing corticosteroids and 39% for complying with instructions for daily peak flowmeter use.[47,48] Several reasons for physician nonadherence to the NAEPP guidelines include time and staff limitations for delivery of recommendations, low reimbursement for visits that provide patient education and medication monitoring, low self-efficacy among clinicians for correctly dosing anti-inflammatory medications and teaching peak flowmeter use,[49] lack of time for education specific to guideline components that involve intensive teaching and counseling,[48] low self-efficacy about counseling for smoking cessation, and clinical inertia or the failure to change therapy when the disease is uncontrolled.[50] Other reasons for nonadherence to guidelines are based in part on provider beliefs, including lack of agreement with safety of long-term corticosteroid use (concerns of cushingoid effects, osteoporosis, growth stunting, cataract development),[47] underestimation by clinicians of children's asthma severity,[13,51] difficulty convincing parents to administer ICSs when they are concerned about side effects,[47] and language barriers in families with English as a second language who may be unable to understand proper medication dosage and administration. In summary, most pediatric providers are aware of the national asthma guidelines and have access to a copy of the guidelines, yet adherence to specific guideline components remains low.

Recommendations to improve access to quality medical care

- Provide alternative health care sites for inner-city children with asthma through school-based asthma programs and community or mobile health care clinics when available.
- Enroll patients into comprehensive disease-management or case-management programs that provide transportation, appointment reminders, and electronic communication with the patient's health care provider to improve the quality of care and monitor asthma status on a regular basis.
- Encourage endorsement of national asthma guidelines by local pediatric professional organizations (American Academy of Pediatrics, National Association of

Pediatric Nurse Practitioners and Nurses, and National Association of School Health Nurses) to improve pediatric health care provider awareness and encourage more use of national asthma guidelines.[9,47,48]

- Provide practical workshops for health care providers, parents, and children to provide hands-on experience with asthma devices, medications, and smoking-cessation counseling.

Psychosocial Factors

Several psychosocial factors are also known to create barriers to preventive care for children with asthma. In particular, caregiver psychological symptoms and life stress related to residence in low-income, inner-city communities negatively influence decisions about asthma self-management and increase asthma morbidity through treatment nonadherence and unnecessary use of health care.[52–56] Both caregiver anxiety and depressive symptoms are associated with poor asthma outcomes,[57,58] but research with inner-city populations increasingly suggests that caregiver depression is a particularly strong predictor of child asthma attacks,[59] ED visits,[60] and hospitalizations.[61] Even when the child's asthma severity is taken into account, caregivers with high levels of depressive symptoms are 30% more likely to report an ED visit by their child than those with low symptomatology.[62]

It is well established that successful asthma self-management requires the caregiver to possess both skill competencies and focused attention to carefully assess and monitor the child's symptoms, administer the correct dosage of preventive medication and stepped-up therapy when needed, and be cognizant of environmental hazards such as mold, rodent infestation, and dust.[44,63] However, depressive symptoms may reduce the caregiver's capacity for the quick and critical thinking that is essential to proper decision making regarding asthma management and health care utilization.[64,65] The clouded judgment may in turn result in avoidable ED and urgent care visits.

Life stress associated with inner-city residence similarly creates barriers to preventive care by disrupting asthma self-management activities.[66] Intimate partner violence (IPV), one example of life stress, is related to poorer health outcomes. The relationship between IPV and asthma in children was examined using the Behavioral Risk Factor Surveillance System survey conducted in 10 US states/territories. Women who experienced IPV at any point in their lifetime were significantly more likely to report that their children ever had or currently have asthma, compared with women who had never experienced IPV.[67]

Both acute (eg, exposure to violence) and chronic (eg, housing instability, poverty) stressors divert attention away from monitoring the child's symptoms and administering controlling medicine.[68] Simply stated, inner-city, low-income caregivers mobilize sparse resources to support "the family's daily survival and future stability".[69(p706)] Adverse social conditions create a barrier to preventive care when a caregiver's physical, financial, and psychological resources are consumed in their efforts to ensure the safety and well-being of the family unit, leaving little time or energy for proper asthma self-management. In summary, symptoms of caregiver depression and life stress may erode the caregiver's ability to perform asthma self-management behaviors as prescribed by the NHLBI, leading to increased asthma morbidity, health care use, and cost.

Recommendations to improve psychosocial challenges

- Provide regular screening of caregiver depression in clinical encounters with child asthma, with referrals to community mental health treatment providers for follow-up care.

- Provide screening for IPV during child asthma encounters, and make appropriate referrals to mental health treatment and community resources to address IPV.
- Caregivers of inner-city minority children with asthma may benefit from counseling strategies to help them cope with contemporary life stressors associated with poverty.[70]

Environmental Factors: Home and Neighborhood Characteristics

Physical and psychosocial aspects of the environment, in both the home and neighborhood, play a significant role in pediatric asthma morbidity. Children in rural environments are at lower risk of asthma compared with children in urban environments.[71] In inner-city environments air pollution is one significant factor, and the home serves as another primary source of allergen and irritant exposures for children, contributing to an increased sensitization to allergens.[72] Allergen sensitivity and exposure are associated with increased asthma morbidity, particularly in sensitized individuals with asthma.[73] The factors associated with this increased sensitization are often related to poverty and poor housing conditions in inner cities, and low-income children are more frequently exposed to environmental triggers,[74] including high levels of indoor allergens,[75] in comparison with children who are not poor. Substandard housing conditions result in exposure to high cockroach and mouse allergen levels,[76] dust mites, and mold related to water and roof leaks. Increased moisture in the home not only augments mold growth but provides a rich environment for dust-mite proliferation. A recent study that pooled allergen, housing conditions, and other data from 9 asthma studies found that high levels of cockroach allergen were associated with cracks or holes in walls, high dust-mite allergen levels with mold odors, and mouse allergen levels with signs of rodents.[77] Furthermore, water leaks and below-average housekeeping was associated with high levels of cockroach allergen. Increased moisture in the home not only augments mold growth but provides a rich environment for dust-mite proliferation. Without pest management, these infestations result in high allergen load in the home, resulting in an increased risk of asthma exacerbation. These high indoor exposures are supported by observations in the authors' current cohort of 300 inner-city children with asthma who reported high levels of rodent and cockroach exposure (mice: 46%; cockroach infestation: 28%) (see **Table 1**).

Other indoor exposures include nitrogen dioxide associated with the use of gas stoves, and exposure to second-hand smoke (SHS). Both indoor exposure to nitrogen dioxide and SHS are associated with negative respiratory effects in asthma.[78] In a recent study of 469 families of children with asthma in a large city, gas stoves were present in 88% of the homes and the median level of indoor nitrogen dioxide was high.[78] This higher level of nitrogen dioxide was related to lower peak flow levels among the children during the colder months.[78] Another prevalent indoor exposure for children is SHS. Of note, between 40% and 67% of inner-city children with asthma reside in a dwelling with at least 1 smoker,[74] which has important implications for children living in substandard housing with poor ventilation. Objective evidence of SHS exposure in a large study of children with asthma reported that the median level of cotinine/creatinine, a biomarker for SHS exposure, was 42.4 ng/mg in children living in homes with a smoker, compared with 18.0 ng/mg in children not residing with a smoker.[78] The authors' data confirm the high prevalence of SHS exposure in inner-city children with asthma, with more than half (59%) of the children residing with a smoker in their home (see **Table 1**).

Besides the physical home environment, psychosocial aspects of neighborhoods and communities influence asthma morbidity. Even though some communities may share low SHS and environmental exposures, such as poor housing or high outdoor pollution, they may not share excess asthma morbidity.[68,79–81] This paradox has resulted in studies examining the role of psychosocial factors within neighborhoods to help explain these differences. For example, researchers have found that individual perceptions of stressors related to living in high-risk neighborhoods and actual community-level indicators are also significantly related to asthma morbidity. Community-level stressors include poverty, unemployment or underemployment, limited social capital, and high exposure to crime and violence.[81] Exposure to community violence is one specific factor related to asthma morbidity. Caretakers of children with asthma and who were exposed to community violence reported more lost sleep and symptom days among their children.[82] In a recent longitudinal study of children with asthma younger than 10 years and residing in Chicago, community violence was also associated with increased asthma risk, although it did not fully explain asthma risk when controlling for individual-level and other neighborhood-level factors.[83]

On the other hand, protective factors at the community level have been described. Cagney and colleagues,[79] for example, studied the paradox of foreign-born Latinos having a respiratory health advantage if they lived in an enclave of other foreign-born Latinos. The explanation for this protective advantage was described as the sense of cohesiveness or collective efficacy present in the community. This level of trust and attachment within a community may be protective for families who feel a sense of cohesiveness and know they can rely on neighbors for assistance if their child has asthma symptoms.[68]

Recommendations to improve physical and neighborhood factors

- Assist families to identify specific allergen triggers for their child, including awareness of both indoor and outdoor allergens and air-pollutant exposures. Provide individualized and comprehensive education about simple household preventive measures such as use of mousetraps, cockroach bait, and repair of water leaks to avoid mold exposure.
- Provide smoking-cessation resources to families with a smoker in the home. National Quitline 1-800-Quit Now.
- Families living in substandard housing may benefit from referral and counseling strategies to help them seek alternative living conditions.
- Assess for exposure to violence; referral to stress-reduction program or to programs that provide counseling to those exposed to violence.
- Promote social cohesion in communities and build social capital (ie, connections within and between social networks) to create better living conditions to improve health.

Cost of Challenges to Providing Preventive Care to Inner-City Children with Asthma

Costs create challenges, with respect to asthma generally and preventive care specifically, in several ways. First, asthma is costly for families. A recent report indicated that the mean out-of-pocket costs for medication related to asthma was $151 for children younger than 5 years and just slightly higher ($154) for children ages 5 to 18.[84] Another study, this time focusing on families of children with asthma in which an adult is employed, found that children having asthma was associated with higher employee costs (health care, prescriptions, sick leave, and short-term disability), and the children's health care ($862) and prescription ($534) spending.[85] With a 20% copayment (common in many insurance policies), the combination of health care and prescriptions for children would result in approximately $280 of additional out-of-pocket costs per year for the family.

A key in interpreting these results is to recognize that these costs are not a small amount for families in difficult economic situations and that asthma in general (and uncontrolled asthma specifically) is associated with poverty.[1] The resources required for routine asthma care compete with other uses of familial resources, including child care for other children and a variety of costs to help improve the environment. For

Table 2
Summary of recommendations by challenge

Challenge	Recommendations
Caregiver and family attitudes and beliefs about asthma care	Identify and discuss parental attitudes, beliefs, and worries about medications Teach parents and school-age children specific and nonspecific symptoms of asthma, and identify child-symptom descriptors for parents and teachers to understand Monitor younger and newly diagnosed children with asthma more frequently, owing to evolving ability to recognize asthma symptoms
Lack of access to quality medical care	Provide alternative health care sites such as school-based asthma programs, community or mobile health care clinics when available Enroll patients into comprehensive disease-management or case-management programs Encourage endorsement of guidelines by local pediatric professional organizations (American Academy of Pediatrics, National Association of Pediatric Nurse Practitioners and Nurses, and National Association of School Health Nurses) to improve pediatric health care provider awareness and use of national asthma guidelines Provide practical workshops to provide hands-on experience with asthma devices, medications, smoking-cessation counseling, and models of asthma care
Psychosocial factors	Regular screening of caregiver depression in child asthma clinical encounters, with referrals to community mental health treatment providers for follow-up care Caregivers of inner-city minority children with asthma may benefit from counseling strategies to help them cope with contemporary life stressors associated with poverty
Environmental factors	Assist families to identify specific allergen triggers for their child. Provide individualized and comprehensive education about simple household preventive measures such as use of mousetraps, cockroach bait, and repair of water leaks to avoid mold exposure Provide smoking-cessation resources to families with smokers in the home. National Quitline 1-800-Quit Now. Families living in substandard housing may benefit from referral and counseling strategies to help them seek alternative living conditions Assess for exposure to violence; referral to stress-reduction program or to programs that provide counseling to those exposed to violence Promote social cohesion in communities and build social capital (ie, connections within and between social networks) to create better living conditions to improve health

example, extermination for mice and cockroaches, air cleaners in the child's bedroom, and mattress covers for dust-mite prevention are all nonnegligible expenses and are usually not covered by insurance. These preventive activities may be given even lower priority than preventive medications, as the impact is apparent only in the longer term, and individuals with limited financial resources tend to focus on the use of resources with the most immediate outcomes.

SUMMARY AND IMPLICATIONS

Preventive asthma care for inner-city children is challenging because of multiple health care system/organizational, caregiver and family, health care provider, psychosocial, and environmental factors that negatively affect preventive care (**Table 2**). Several recommendations to help minimize the barriers to preventive asthma care are suggested for pediatric nurses who care for these high-risk children across multiple settings. To enhance asthma self-management and reduce barriers to preventive care, clinical work with this population must extend beyond screening for traditional environmental risk factors (eg, allergens and irritants) to also include comprehensive assessment of caregiver attitudes and beliefs, caregiver stressors, and targeted referrals for modifiable psychosocial stressors that influence caregiver behaviors. Furthermore, pediatric health care providers can monitor the level of stress, anxiety, or depression, and recommend either management strategies or links to services that might help patients and caregivers to manage these stressors. Because exposure to allergens and irritants plays a significant role in asthma morbidity, families may need assistance with identification of specific allergen triggers and awareness of indoor and outdoor exposures, and their effects on children with asthma. Effective remediation of allergen and pollutant exposure involves individualized and comprehensive family education about household preventive measures such as use of mousetraps and cockroach bait, and repair of water leaks to avoid mold exposure. Lastly, endorsement of national guidelines by local pediatric professional organizations to improve awareness in pediatric health care providers is recommended, along with the use of national asthma guidelines.

REFERENCES

1. Akinbami LJ, Moorman JE, Bailey C, et al. Trends in asthma prevalence, health care use and mortality in the United States, 2001-2010. NCHS Data Brief 2012;94:1–7.
2. Akinbami LJ, Moorman JE, Garbe PL, et al. Status of childhood asthma in the United States, 1980-2007. Pediatrics 2009;123(S3):S131–45.
3. Akinbami L. The state of childhood asthma, United States, 1980-2005. Centers for Disease Control and Prevention National Center for Health Statistics. Adv Data 2006 Dec 12;(381):1–24.
4. Akinbami LJ, Moorman JE, Liu X. Asthma prevalence, health care use and mortality: United States, 2005-2009. Natl Health Stat Report 2011;12(32):1–14.
5. Diaz T, Sturm T, Matte T, et al. Medication use among children with asthma in East Harlem. Pediatrics 2000;105(6):1188–93.
6. Ortega AN, Gergen PJ, Paltiel AD, et al. Impact of site of care, race, and Hispanic ethnicity on medication use for childhood asthma. Pediatrics 2002; 109(1):E1.
7. Centers for Disease Control and Prevention (CDC). Vital signs: asthma prevalence, disease characteristics, and self-management education—United States, 2001-2009. MMWR Morb Mortal Wkly Rep 2011;60(17):547–52.

8. Bethell CD, Kogan MD, Strickland BB, et al. A National and State profile of leading health problems and heath care quality for US children: key insurance disparities and across-state variations. Academic Pediatrics 2011;11(Suppl 3): S22–33.

9. Finkelstein JA, Lozano P, Shulruff R, et al. Self-reported physician practices for children with asthma: are national guidelines followed? Pediatrics 2000;106(Suppl 4): 886–96.

10. Crain EF, Weiss KB, Fagan MJ. Pediatric asthma care in US emergency departments. Current practice in the context of the National Institutes of Health Guidelines. Arch Pediatr Adolesc Med 1995;149:893–901.

11. Wisnivesky JP, Lorenzo J, Lyn-cook R, et al. Barriers to adherence to asthma management guidelines among inner-city primary care providers. Ann Allergy Asthma Immunol 2008;101:264–70.

12. Van den Berg NJ, Hagmolen W, Nagelkerke AF, et al. What general practitioners and paediatricians think about their patients' asthma. Patient Educ Couns 2005; 59:182–95.

13. Halterman JS, Yoos HL, Kaczorowski JM, et al. Providers underestimate symptom severity among urban children with asthma. Archives of Pediatric and Adolescent Medicine 2002;156:141–6.

14. Butz AM, Tsoukleris M, Donithan M, et al. Patterns of inhaled anti-inflammatory medication use in young underserved children with asthma. Pediatrics 2006; 118:2504–13.

15. Kattan M, Crain EF, Steinbach S, et al. A randomized clinical trial of clinician feedback to improve quality of care for inner-city children with asthma. Pediatrics 2006;117:e1095–103.

16. Gregor MA, Wheeler JR, Stanley RM, et al, Great Lakes Emergency Medical Services for Children Research Network. Caregiver adherence to follow-up after an emergency department visit for common pediatric illnesses: impact on future ED use. Med Care 2009;47(3):326–33.

17. Brousseau D, Dansereau L, Linakis J, et al. Pediatric emergency department utilization within a statewide Medicaid managed care system. Academic Emergency Medicine 2002;9:296–9.

18. Otsuki M, Eakin M, Arceneaux LL, et al. Prospective relationship between maternal depressive symptoms and asthma morbidity among inner-city African American Children. J Pediatr Psychology 2010;35(7):758–67.

19. Turyk ME, Hernandez E, Wright RJ, et al. Stressful life events and asthma in adolescents. Pediatr Allergy Immunol 2008;19(3):255–63.

20. Conn KM, Halterman JS, Fisher SG, et al. Parental beliefs about medications and medication adherence among urban children with asthma. Ambulatory Pediatrics 2005;5:306–10.

21. Bender BG, Bender SE. Patient-identified barriers to asthma treatment adherence: response to interviews, focus groups and questionnaires. Immunol Allergy Clin N Am 2005;25:107–30.

22. Halterman JS, McConnochie KM, Conn KM, et al. A randomized trial of primary care provider prompting to enhance preventive asthma therapy. Arch Pediatr Adolesc Med 2005;159(5):422–7.

23. Flores G, Snowden-Bridon C, Torres S, et al. Urban minority children with asthma: substantial morbidity, compromised quality and access to specialists, and the importance of poverty and specialty care. J Asthma 2009;46:392–8.

24. Juniper EF, Guyatt GH, Feeny DH, et al. Measuring quality of life in the parents and children with asthma. Qual Life Res 1996;5(1):27–34.

25. Horne R, Weinman J. Self-regulation and self-management in asthma: exploring the role of illness perceptions and treatment beliefs in explaining non-adherence to preventer medication. Psychology and Health 2002;17(1):17–32.
26. Butz AM, Halterman JS, Bellin M, et al. Factors associated with caregiver completion of a behavioral intervention for primary care providers and caregivers of urban children with asthma. J Asthma 2012;49(9):977–88. http://dx.doi.org/10.3109/02770903.2012.721435.
27. Yoos HL, Kitzman H, McMullen A, et al. Symptom perception in childhood asthma: how accurate are children and their parents? Journal of Asthma 2003; 40:27–39.
28. Fritz GK, Yeung A, Wamboldt MZ, et al. Conceptual and methodological issues in quantifying perceptual accuracy in childhood asthma. J Pediatr Psychol 1996;21: 153–73.
29. Yoos HL, Kitzman H, McMullen A, et al. The language of breathlessness: do families and health care providers speak the same language when describing asthma symptoms? J Pediatr Health Care 2005;19:197–205.
30. Diette GB, Skinner EA, Markson LE, et al. Consistency of care with national guidelines for children with asthma in managed care. J Pediatrics 2001;138: 59–64.
31. Zorc JJ, Scarfone RJ, Li Y. Predictors of primary care follow-up after a pediatric emergency visits for asthma. J Asthma 2005;42:571–6.
32. Armstrong HE, Ishiki D, Heiman J, et al. Service utilization by black and white clientele in an urban community mental health center. Revised assessment of an old problem. Community Mental Health Journal 1984;20:269–81.
33. Smith SR, Highstein GR, Jaffe DM, et al. Parental impressions of the benefits (pros) and barriers (cons) of follow-up care after an acute emergency department visit for children with asthma. Pediatrics 2002;110:323–30.
34. Smith SR, Jaffe DM, Fisher EB, et al. Improving follow-up for children with asthma after an acute emergency department visit. J Pediatr 2004;145:772–7.
35. Baren JM, Boudreaux ED, Brenner BE, et al. Randomized controlled trial of emergency department interventions to improve primary care follow-up for patients with acute asthma. Chest 2006;129:257–65.
36. Teach SJ, Crain EF, Quint DM, et al. Improved asthma outcomes in a high-morbidity pediatric population. Arch Pediatr Adolesc Med 2006;160:535–41.
37. Meischke H, Lozano P, Zhou C, et al. Engagement in "My Child's Asthma", an incentive web-based pediatric asthma management intervention. Int J Medical Informatics 2011;80(11):765–74.
38. Onyirimba F, Apter A, Reisine S, et al. Direct clinician-to-patient feedback discussion of inhaled steroid use: its effect on adherence. Ann Allergy Asthma Immunol 2003;90:411–5.
39. Halterman JS, Szilagyi P, Fisher S, et al. A randomized controlled trial to improve care for urban children with asthma: results of the School-Based Asthma Therapy trial. Arch Pediatr Adolesc Med 2011;165:262–8.
40. Halterman JS, Sauer J, Fagnano M, et al. Working toward a sustainable system of asthma care: development of the school-based preventive asthma care technology (SB-PACT) Trial. J Asthma 2012;49(4):395–400.
41. Bollinger ME, Morphew T, Mullins CD. The Breathmobile program: a good investment for underserved children with asthma. Ann Allergy Asthma Immunol 2010; 105:274–81.
42. Douglas JM. Mobile dental vans: planning considerations and productivity. J Public Health Dentistry 2005;65(2):110–3.

43. Jones CA, Clement LT, Hanley-Lopez J, et al. The Breathmobile Program: structure, implementation and evolution of a large-scale, urban, pediatric asthma disease management program. Dis Manag 2005;8:205–22.
44. U.S. Department of Health and Human Services (USDHHS). The National Asthma Education and Prevention Program. Expert Panel Report 3 (EPR3): Guidelines for the diagnosis and management of asthma. NIH Publication No. 07-4051, August 2007.
45. Celano MP, Linzer JF, Demi A, et al. Treatment adherence among low-income, African American children with persistent asthma. J Asthma 2010;47:317–22.
46. Butz AM, Walker J, Land CL, et al. Improving asthma communication in high-risk children. J Asthma 2007;44:739–45.
47. Cabana MD, Ebel BE, Cooper-Patrick L, et al. Barriers pediatricians face when using asthma practice guidelines. Arch Pediatr Adolesc Med 2000;154:685–93.
48. Cabana MD, Rand CS, Becher OJ, et al. Reasons for pediatrician nonadherence to asthma guidelines. Arch Pediatr Adolesc Med 2001;155:1057–62.
49. Cabana MD, Flores G. The role of clinical practice guidelines in enhancing quality and reducing racial/ethnic disparities in pediatrics. Paediatric Respiratory Reviews 2002;3:52–8.
50. Phillips LS, Branch WT Jr, Cook CB. Clinical inertia. Ann Intern Med 2001;135: 825–34.
51. Revicki D, Weiss KB. Clinical assessment of asthma symptom control: review of current assessment instruments. J Asthma 2006;43:481–7.
52. Wolf JM, Miller GE, Chen E. Parent psychological states predict changes in inflammatory markers in children with asthma and healthy children. Brain Behav Immun 2008;22:433–41.
53. Mangan JM, Wittich AR, Gerald LB. The potential for reducing asthma disparities through improved family and social function and modified health behaviors. Chest 2007;132:789S–801S.
54. Shalowitz MU, Mijanovich T, Berry CA, et al. Context matters: a community-based study of maternal mental health, life stressors, social support, and children's asthma. Pediatrics 2006;117:e940–8.
55. Strunk RC, Ford JG, Taggart V. Reducing disparities in asthma care: priorities for research—National Heart, Lung, and Blood Institute Workshop Report. J Allergy Clin Immunol 2002;109:229–37.
56. Szabo A, Mezei G, Kovari E, et al. Depressive symptoms amongst asthmatic children's caregivers. Pediatr Allergy Immunol 2010;21:e667–73.
57. Brown SE, Gan V, Jeffress J, et al. Psychiatric symptomatology and disorders in caregivers of children with asthma. Pediatrics 2006;118:e1715–20.
58. Silver EJ, Warman KL, Stein RE. The relationship of caretaker anxiety to children's asthma morbidity and acute care utilization. J Asthma 2005;42:379–83.
59. Feldman JM, Perez EA, Canino G, et al. The role of caregiver major depression in the relationship between anxiety disorders and asthma attacks in Island Puerto Rican youth and young adults. J Nerv Ment Dis 2011;119:313–8.
60. Lange NE, Bunyavanich S, Silberg JL, et al. Parental psychosocial stress and asthma morbidity in Puerto Rican twins. J Allergy Clin Immunol 2010;127:734–40.
61. Flynn HA, Davis M, Marcus SM, et al. Rates of maternal depression in pediatric emergency department and relationship to child service utilization. Gen Hosp Psychiatry 2004;26:316–22.
62. Bartlett SJ, Kolodner K, Butz AM, et al. Maternal depressive symptoms and emergency department use among inner-city children with asthma. Arch Pediatr Adolesc Med 2001;155:347–53.

63. Martinez KG, Perez EA, Ramirez R, et al. The role of caregivers' depressive symptoms and asthma beliefs on asthma outcomes among low-income Puerto Rican children. J Asthma 2009;46:136–41.
64. Bartlett S, Krishnan J, Riekert K, et al. Maternal depressive symptoms and adherence to therapy in inner-city children with asthma. Pediatr 2004;113:229–37.
65. DiMatteo MR, Lepper HS, Croghan TW. Depression is a risk factor for noncompliance with medical treatment. Arch Intern Med 2000;160:2101–7.
66. Quinn K, Kaufman JS, Siddiqi A, et al. Stress and the city: housing stressors are associated with respiratory health among low socioeconomic status Chicago children. J Urban Health 2010b;87:688–702.
67. Breiding MJ, Ziembroski JS. The relationship between intimate partner violence and children's asthma in 10 US states/territories. Pediatr Allergy Immunol 2011; 22(1 Pt 2):e95–100.
68. Quinn K, Kaufman JS, Siddiqi A, et al. Parent perceptions of neighborhood stressors are associated with general health and child respiratory health among low-income urban families. J Asthma 2010a;47:281–9.
69. Yinusa-Nyahkoon LS, Cohn ES, Cortes DE, et al. Ecological barriers and social forces in childhood asthma management: examining routines of African American families living in the inner city. J Asthma 2010;47:701–10.
70. Bellin MH, Kub J, Frick K, et al. Stress and quality of life in caregivers of inner-city minority children with poorly controlled asthma. J Pediatric Health Care 2013; 27(2).
71. Priftis KN, Mantzouranis EC, Antrhacopoulos MB. Asthma symptoms and airway narrowing in children growing up in an urban versus rural environment. J Asthma 2009;46:244–51.
72. Eggleston PA. The environment and asthma in US inner cities. Chest 2007; 132(Suppl 5):782S–8S.
73. Sheehan WJ, Sheehan MD, Rangsithienchal PA, et al. Pest and allergen exposure and abatement in inner-city asthma: a Work Group Report of the American Academy of Allergy, Asthma & Immunology Indoor Allergy/Air Pollution Committee. J Allergy Clin Immunol 2010;125:575–81.
74. Gruchalla RS, Pongracic J, Plaut M, et al. Inner-city Asthma Study: relationship among sensitivity, allergen exposure, and asthma morbidity. J Allergy Clin Immunol 2005;115(3):478–85.
75. National Research Council "Front Matter". Clearing the air: asthma and indoor air exposures. Washington, DC: National Academy Press; 2000.
76. Krieger J, Jacobs DE, Ashley PJ, et al. Housing interventions and control of asthma-related indoor biologic agents: a review of evidence. J Public Health Management Practice 2010;16(5):S11–20.
77. Wilson J, Dixon SL, Breysse P, et al. Housing and allergens: a pooled analysis of nine US cities. Environ Research 2010;110:189–98.
78. Kattan M, Gergen PJ, Eggleston P. Health effects of indoor nitrogen dioxide and passive smoking on urban asthmatic children. J Allergy Clin Immunol 2007; 120(3):618–24.
79. Cagney KA, Browning CR, Wallace DM. The Latino paradox in neighborhood context: the case of asthma and other respiratory conditions. Am J Public Health 2007;97:919–25.
80. Sandel M, Wright RJ. When home is where the stress is: expanding the dimensions of housing that influence asthma morbidity. Arch Dis Child 2006;91:942–8.
81. Wright RJ, Subramanian SV. Advancing a multilevel framework for epidemiologic research on asthma disparities. Chest 2007;132(Suppl 5):757S–69S.

82. Wright RJ, Mitchell H, Visness CM, et al. Community violence and asthma morbidity: the inner-city asthma study. Am J Public Health 2004;94(4):625–32.
83. Sternthal MJ, Jun HJ, Earls F, et al. Community violence and urban childhood asthma: a multilevel analysis. Eur Respir J 2010;36(6):1400–9.
84. Karaca-Mandic P, Jena AB, Joyce GF, et al. Out-of-pocket medication costs and use of medications and health care services among children with asthma. JAMA 2012;307(12):1284–91.
85. Kleinman NL, Brook RA, Ramachandran S. An employer perspective on annual employee and dependent costs for pediatric asthma. Ann Allergy Asthma and Immunol 2009;103:114–20.

Pediatric Obesity and Asthma Quality of Life

Barbara Velsor-Friedrich, PhD, RN[a],*,
Lisa K. Militello, MSN, MPH, CPNP[b], Joanne Kouba[c],
Patrick R. Harrison, BS, MA[d], Amy Manion, PhD, RN, CPNP[e],
Rita Doumit, PhD, RN[f]

KEYWORDS

- Asthma • Obesity • Youth • Quality of life

KEY POINTS

- The literature to date highlights existing gaps and provides several outlets for future research.
- The comorbid prevalence of obesity and asthma in youth is clearly an area requiring additional research.
- It is evident that health disparities exist for both asthma and obesity, especially in both Hispanic and African American youth.
- It is suggested that for these at-risk populations, weight-management and weight-reduction education should be included in every health-related visit.
- In addition, because of the negative effect of asthma and obesity on quality of life, tools such as the Pediatric Asthma Quality of Life Questionnaire should be used at every asthma evaluation visit and quality-of-life issues discussed, and incorporated into the asthma treatment plan.

BACKGROUND AND SIGNIFICANCE
Adult Obesity

The phenomenon of unhealthy weight status in the United States has captured the attention of health professionals and the public alike. Dramatic increases in body mass index (BMI; weight in kilograms divided by height in meters squared, ie, kg/m^2)

[a] Niehoff School of Nursing, Loyola University Chicago, Granada Center Room 355B, 1032 West Loyola Avenue, Chicago, IL 60626, USA; [b] College of Nursing, Arizona State University, 500 North 3rd Street, Phoenix, AZ 85004-0698, USA; [c] Niehoff School of Nursing, Loyola University Chicago, 2160 South First Avenue, Maywood, IL 60153, USA; [d] Department of Psychology, Loyola University Chicago, 1032 West Loyola Avenue, Coffee Hall, Chicago, IL 60626, USA; [e] College of Nursing, 600 South Paulina Avenue Suite 440, Amour Academic Center, Chicago, IL 60612, USA; [f] University of Lebanon Beirut Campus
* Corresponding author.
E-mail address: bvelsor@luc.edu

Nurs Clin N Am 48 (2013) 259–270
http://dx.doi.org/10.1016/j.cnur.2013.01.011
0029-6465/13/$ – see front matter © 2013 Elsevier Inc. All rights reserved.

have been reported through public health surveillance programs such as the National Health and Nutrition Examination Survey (NHANES) starting in the 1970s to the 1990s for both adults and youth, making obesity and overweight common conditions in the United States. According to the most recent NHANES reports, using data from 2009 to 2010, age-adjusted obesity prevalence for adults is 35.7% and overweight prevalence for this group is 33.1%. In other words, 68.8% of adults in the United States have a BMI greater than is considered healthy.[1]

The burden of high BMI is not equally distributed among all segments of the adult population. Analysis of NHANES trends from 1999 to 2010 suggests that significant increases in obesity prevalence have occurred for white, non-Hispanic black, and Mexican American men, and non-Hispanic black and Mexican American women.[1]

Obesity in Youth

The obesity phenomenon in youth parallels that of adults in the United States. Childhood obesity has tripled in the last 4 decades. Current estimates are that 16.9% of youth between 2 and 19 years of age are obese (BMI ≥95th percentile for age) and 14.9% are overweight (BMI between the 85th and 94th percentile for age), which results in a total of 31.8% of youth in the United States meeting criteria for unhealthy weight.[2] As a child's age increases, so does their likelihood of being overweight or obese, as shown in **Table 1**. Preschool children aged 2 to 5 years have lower odds (0.58 for males; 0.62 for females) of obesity compared with adolescents aged 12 to 19 years.[2] Similar to disparities in adults, the burden of excess weight is more prevalent in black and Hispanic youth, and in both genders, as shown in **Table 1**. For youth combined between 2 and 19 years old, males have a significantly higher prevalence of obesity (18.6%) than females (15%)[2]; this holds true for white but not Hispanic or non-Hispanic black youth.

Youth Obesity and Asthma

The prevalence of both asthma and obesity has increased dramatically over the last several decades, which has led to an increase in the number of studies examining the relationship between these 2 variables.[3,4] However, despite the increased interest in these comorbidities, much of the research in this area has focused on adults.[3,5–7]

A study examining the prevalence of obesity among adults, using data from the NHANES I, II, and III, showed that adults with asthma are far more likely to be obese than adults without asthma.[3] In a retrospective study of 143 adult individuals aged 18 to 88 years, the prevalence of obesity increased along with increasing asthma severity in adults.[5] Furthermore, the results showed that females with asthma were significantly more overweight than males, with a mean BMI of 35.9 versus 32.14

Table 1
Prevalence of high body mass index (BMI; ≥85th percentile) in United States youth: both genders combined for selected groups

BMI ≥85th Percentile	2–19 Years Old	2–5 Years Old	6–11 Years Old	12–19 Years Old
All racial/ethnic groups	31.8	26.7	32.6	33.6
Non-Hispanic white	27.9	23.8	27.6	30.0
Mexican American	39.4	33.3	39	43.4
Non-Hispanic black	39.1	41.8	42.7	41.2

Data from Ogden CL, Carroll MD, Kit BK, et al. Prevalence of obesity and trends in body mass index among US children and adolescents, 1999–2010. JAMA 2012;307(5):483–90.

(P = .01). These findings suggest that obesity may be a potentially modifiable risk factor for asthma.[5]

The relationship between asthma and high BMI has also been examined in youth. Much of this research has focused on low-income urban and minority populations, owing to the higher prevalence of asthma and obesity in these groups. In a sample (N = 171) of predominantly Hispanic (78%) youth, 45.9% of those with asthma were overweight or obese compared with 30.2% of those without asthma who were overweight or obese (P = .04).[8] It was unclear whether exercise-induced asthma symptoms resulted in exercise avoidance and obesity, or if obesity exacerbated asthma symptoms with exercise. Belamarich and colleagues[9] examined inner-city children with asthma and determined that there was a higher incidence of obesity in Latino study subjects. In addition, obese children with asthma used more asthma medications, wheezed more, and had a greater proportion of unscheduled visits to the emergency department (ED).

A cross-sectional study using data from the 1988 to 1994 NHANES documented that 2 of the highest-risk groups for developing asthma were children older than 10 years with a BMI greater than or equal to the 85th percentile, and children with a parental history of asthma who were 10 years or younger and of African American ethnicity.[10] A subsequent study of NHANES data between 1999 and 2006 included 16,074 youth between the ages of 2 and 19 years.[11] The odds of asthma for those categorized as overweight and obese were 1.32 and 1.68, respectively, after adjustment for age, survey period, race/ethnicity, gender, and other social factors. Overweight and obesity were also associated with a higher likelihood for an asthma attack, visits to the ED, wheezing episodes, missed school, or ambulatory care visit in the last year. Limitations of studies based on NHANES data are the cross-sectional study design and the self-reporting of asthma.

A large cross-sectional study examined relationships between current asthma diagnosis, weight status, and race/ethnicity using information from 681,122 electronic medical records of youth in the Kaiser Permanente health system between 2007 and 2009.[12] The prevalence of current physician-diagnosed asthma with current medication use was 10.9%. Black youth were more likely to have asthma than non-Hispanic white youth (odds ratio = 1.93). When asthma diagnosis was examined for various weight categories, a dose-response relationship was noted, with increasing odds of asthma for those who were classified as overweight, obese, or extremely obese reported as 1.22, 1.37, and 1.68, respectively (P<.001 for trend).

When the data were further stratified by race/ethnicity and weight status, differences were noted. The dose-response relationship between weight status and risk of asthma was most pronounced in the Native American/Alaskan population, with odds of asthma for the extremely obese being 3.65 times that of asthma for normal-weight Native Americans/Alaskan youth. However, because of the small sample size (n = 610), statistical significance was not established. This dose-response relationship was statistically significant for the white sample, with odds of 1.3, 1.47, and 1.93 for those who were overweight, obese, and extremely obese in comparison with normal weight. This relationship was also identified in black youth, although with smaller and narrower odds. Also interesting was that the odds for asthma with increasing weight status was less in Hispanic youth with high BMI than in white youth with high BMI, though still higher than in normal-weight Hispanic youth. Researchers also found that those with extreme obesity were 18% more likely to use oral corticosteroids (P<.001), and 9% more likely to use inhaled corticosteroids (P<.001) than normal-weight youth. Extremely obese youth with asthma made 274 more ambulatory care visits per 1000 youth (P<.001) and 23 more ED visits (P<.001) than normal-weight youth with asthma. Strengths of this study included physician-diagnosed asthma and the large sample.

International studies report similar findings. A study conducted in Taiwan examined the relationship between asthma, lung function, and BMI in more than 15,000 school-aged children. The prevalence of asthma increased as BMI increased in both males and females.[13] A similar result was found in a study conducted in Nova Scotia, Canada, which examined 3804 students 10 to 11 years of age. Controlling for socio-economic factors, there was a linear association between BMI and asthma, with a 6% increase in prevalence per unit increase of BMI.[14]

The consistency of the studies noted offer promising support of the correlation between high BMI and asthma. However, many used a cross-sectional design aiding in hypothesis generation but not adding to insights about causation.

The systematic review of Noal and colleagues[15] provides insights into the temporal relationship between BMI and asthma and the causal path. Ten longitudinal studies examined the relationship between weight status in early childhood and the development of asthma in adolescence. With one exception, all studies reported sample sizes greater than 1000. The majority (8 of 10) of the studies reported a positive association between overweight or obesity in early childhood and the development of asthma in adolescence. For example, Mannino and colleagues[16] followed 4393 asthma-free children for up to 14 years. Analysis of the data showed that boys with a BMI at or greater than the 85th percentile at age 2 to 3 years and boys with a BMI consistently at or above the 85th percentile were at higher risk for subsequent asthma development. Three of the studies reported in the systematic review by Noal and colleagues[15] reported higher risk for females, 3 studies reported higher risk for males, and 2 reported that the relationship was independent of gender. Although this review provides support for the causative role of high BMI in asthma incidence because of its longitudinal study design, the mechanisms for this relationship are still unclear. Proposed hypotheses have included a mechanical effect of obesity on respiratory function, the role of obesity in fueling inflammatory responses leading to asthma and/or obesity-induced immune changes that trigger genetic or hormonal pathways for asthma. Environmental factors that promote obesity, such as sedentary lifestyle, diet, and low birth weight, may also promote asthma development.[15] Clearly the rising incidence of asthma and obesity, and their combined impact on youth's quality of life (QOL), requires additional investigation.

REVIEW OF THE LITERATURE
Pediatric Asthma Quality of Life

The need to address QOL issues in chronically ill youth has become a priority in the United States.[17] There are several reasons for examining QOL in adolescents with asthma as a unique group distinct from young children and adults. Adolescence is a period of emergence of independent thinking and behavior which, along with various stressors, such as peer pressure, may affect the interpretation of asthma symptoms and adherence to prescribed asthma therapy.[18–20] This concept was supported in a study by Bruzzese and colleagues,[20] which found that early adolescents' asthma self-management was suboptimal. Although they perceive themselves to have greater responsibility for managing their asthma, early adolescents did less to care for their asthma, suggesting they may be given responsibility for asthma care prematurely.

Clinicians and researchers routinely use QOL as an indicator of successful management of asthma in youth. Measures of QOL are thought to indicate how much an adolescent's illness interferes with daily life and how well the teenager is adapting to his or her illness across several areas of functioning such as social, emotional, and physical.

A systematic review by Everhart and Fiese[21] found that asthma severity was a correlate of QOL in youth with asthma. Youth whose asthma symptoms were not well managed were more likely to experience an impaired level of QOL. Everhart and Fiese[21] concluded that researchers and health care providers basing clinical outcomes on QOL assessments should consider asthma severity in their evaluations.

These findings were supported by another study conducted with 533 Dutch adolescents. Symptom severity affected overall and positive QOL, both directly and indirectly, via coping. The lifestyle restricted by coping strategies and worrying about asthma were associated with poorer overall QOL. The use of the coping strategies–restricted lifestyle, positive reappraisal, and information seeking was related to increased scores on the positive QOL domain, whereas hiding asthma was related to lower scores on the positive QOL domain.[22]

Burkhart and colleagues[18] explored the predictors of QOL among adolescents from the United States and Iceland. Statistically significant predictors of higher asthma QOL were a better rating of overall health ($P<.01$), not having had a severe asthma attack in the last 6 months ($P<.01$), and lower depressive symptoms ($P<.01$). The researchers concluded that interventions designed to decrease depression and prevent asthma exacerbations might improve QOL for adolescents with asthma. In line with this study, Mohangoo and colleagues[23] evaluated health-related QOL (HRQOL) in adolescents with wheezing attacks using self-reported data, and determined independent associations between wheezing attacks and QOL. The presence of at least 4 wheezing attacks during the past year was associated with relevant deficits in QOL.

Another study conducted by Schmier and colleagues[24] evaluated asthma-related activity limitations and productivity losses among children and adolescents (age 4–18 years). Both HRQOL and productivity were significantly lower in patients with inadequately controlled asthma when compared with those with controlled asthma. Inadequately controlled asthma had a significant impact on asthma-specific HRQOL, school productivity and attendance, and work productivity of children and their caregivers.

Bruzzese and colleagues[25] tested the efficacy of an 8-week school-based intervention (Asthma Self-Management for Adolescents, ASMA) on 345 primarily Latino (46%) and African American (31%) high school students (mean age 15.1 years, 70% female) reporting an asthma diagnosis, symptoms of moderate to severe persistent asthma, and use of asthma medication in the last 12 months. Primary outcomes were asthma self-management, symptom frequency, and QOL; secondary outcomes were asthma medical management, school absences, days with activity limitations, and urgent health care use. Participants reported significant increases in confidently managing their asthma; use of controller medication and written treatment plans; fewer night awakenings, days with activity limitation, and school absences due to asthma; improved QOL; and fewer acute care visits, ED visits, and hospitalizations.

The feasibility of a motivational interviewing–based asthma self-management program (5 home visits) was developed and assessed in 37 African American adolescents with asthma (age 10–15 years). The teens had recently been seen in an inner-city ED for asthma symptoms and were prescribed an asthma controller medication.[26,27] Although there were no pre-post differences in adolescent-reported medication adherence, participants did report increased motivation and readiness to adhere to treatment. Teens and their caregivers reported statistically significant increases in their asthma QOL. The findings from this pilot study suggest that motivational interviewing is a feasible and promising approach for increasing medication adherence among inner-city adolescents with asthma, and is worthy of further evaluation in a randomized trial.

Pediatric Asthma, Obesity, and QOL

Although asthma severity has been shown to negatively affect QOL, there has been limited research conducted on the effects of both obesity and asthma on QOL despite the increasing prevalence of both diseases. The few studies that have explored QOL, asthma, and obesity in adults have demonstrated mixed results. A study of 382 adults with asthma discovered that the patients with higher BMIs reported lower QOL scores regardless of asthma severity.[25] Grammer and colleagues[28] studied 352 adults with asthma, 191 of whom were obese. Using the Asthma Quality of Life Questionnaire (AQLQ), results showed that obesity directly correlated with decreased QOL and increased health care utilization as demonstrated by ED/urgent care encounters. A second study using the AQLQ examined more than 900 patients, both adults and children, and found similar results in the adult group; obesity significantly correlated with decreased QOL. However, the researchers found no correlation between AQLQ scores and obesity in the children studied. There was no increase in health care use for either the obese adults or children.[29]

Researchers in Germany compared QOL in children with obesity, asthma/atopic dermatitis, or both, using the German KINDL QOL questionnaire. Among the 3 groups, the results showed lower QOL scores in children with obesity, which improved following obesity treatment.[30]

In another international study, Blandon and colleagues[31] examined 100 obese, overweight, and normal-weight children in Mexico with intermittent or mild persistent asthma. There were significant differences in QOL in the obese asthmatic group ($P<.000$). A third study conducted in the Netherlands by van Gent and colleagues,[32] using the Pediatric Asthma Quality of Life Questionnaire, found children with both asthma and obesity had lower (25%) QOL scores than children with either asthma alone (14%) or obesity alone (1%).

From the review of the literature, there appears to be a relationship between asthma and obesity. However, the exact nature of this relationship has yet to be fully determined.[33] Given the rising prevalence of obesity and asthma, additional studies regarding asthma, obesity, and QOL are warranted in order to better understand the interaction between the two comorbidities. In addition, the mechanism behind the link between asthma and obesity needs to be further investigated. The knowledge gained from further studies will aid in the development of more effective treatments and prevention programs for both asthma and obesity.

School-Based Asthma Education Programs

Coffman and colleagues[34] conducted a systematic review of the literature on school-based asthma education programs for youth aged 4 to 17 years with a clinical diagnosis of asthma or symptoms consistent with asthma. Synthesizing across studies was difficult because the characteristics of interventions and target populations varied widely, as did the outcomes assessed. Most studies that compared asthma education with usual care found that school-based asthma education programs improved knowledge of asthma, self-efficacy, and self-management behaviors. Fewer studies reported favorable effects on QOL, symptom days, symptom nights, and school absences.

More recently other supportive interventions, such as cognitive behavior modification strategies, have been found to be successful in treating children and adolescents with chronic illnesses. Interventions that use behavioral strategies are more effective in supporting change than are solely knowledge-based interventions.[35–37] Coping skills training (CST) is based on social cognitive theory, and stresses the use of adaptive coping methods and problem-solving skills. The goal of CST is to teach children and adolescents personal and social coping skills that can assist them in dealing with potential stressors they encounter in their daily lives and the stress reactions that may result from these situations.[38] The use of such skills can increase a teen's sense of competence and self-efficacy in dealing with a wide range of daily demands and health issues. In the youth population, CST has resulted in decreasing substance abuse,[39] increased social skills and reduction of aggressive behaviors,[40] and a decrease in negative responses to stressors.[41] It has also been used successfully in children with chronic illnesses such as cancer and diabetes[42–44] and in minority youth with diabetes.[45,46]

STUDY BY THE AUTHOR
Purpose

The purpose of this study is to report on the specific effects of childhood obesity and asthma on self-reported asthma QOL, coping, and control of asthma health outcomes in low-income African American teens with asthma. A randomized controlled trial (n = 137) was conducted to evaluate the efficacy of a school-based asthma education/management program on asthma-related QOL and other psychosocial and health outcomes in urban African American teens with asthma. The intervention components and results of the study have been reported in detail elsewhere.[47] In brief, the TEAM program (Teen Education and Asthma Management) is composed of 3 elements: (1) asthma education; (2) CST; and (3) nurse practitioner re-enforcement visits.

Methods

Students were recruited from 5 African American dominant urban high schools. Approximately 94% of students and their families received public assistance. Student assent and parent/guardian assent was obtained. Randomization occurred by school because individual randomization within schools could lead to contamination. Students in both the treatment and control groups attended 2 asthma education sessions (group format), 3 educational re-enforcement sessions (group sessions), and an individual clinic visit with the TEAM nurse practitioner at baseline and at the end of program.

Students in the intervention group participated in CST. Five CST sessions were offered once a week during the extended homeroom period for 45 minutes. A makeup session was offered at the end of the fifth session. The following skills were taught: (1) social problem solving; (2) effective communication; (3) managing stress; (4) conflict resolution; and (5) cognitive restructuring (guided self-dialogue). At each session a skill was taught and then students were asked to role-play the skill within an asthma-based scenario. Each week the previous skill was reviewed and the new skills were taught in the same manner. Data were collected at baseline and at 2, 6, and 12 months.

Measures

The Parent Questionnaire was completed by the student's parent/guardian and supplies information regarding demographics and the adolescent's current and prior asthma health status.

The Pediatric Asthma Quality of Life Questionnaire[48] is a 23-item, 7-point Likert-scale instrument that assesses both physiologic and emotional functional impairments experienced by children and adolescents. There are 3 subscales: symptoms experienced (10 items), activity limitation (5 items), and emotional functional (8 items). Total scale α values ranged from 0.93 to 0.94 across all time periods.

Coping was measured using the Kid Cope,[49,50] a 17-item inventory designed to assess 10 cognitive and behavioral strategies used by adolescents. These strategies include distraction, social withdrawal, cognitive restructuring, self-criticism, blaming others, problem-solving, emotional regulation, wishful thinking, social support, and resignation. Total scale α values ranged from 0.73 to 0.86 across time periods.

Control of Asthma Health Outcomes was operationally defined as according to the National Asthma Education and Prevention Program guidelines.[51] For this study, well-controlled was defined as meeting all of the following criteria: mean peak flow reading in the green zone, asthma symptom frequency less than 2 days a week, asthma symptom frequency less than 2 nights per month, and the use of asthma rescue medicine less than 2 days per week.

Overweight and obesity were operationally defined per the Centers for Disease Control criterion and plotted on age-appropriate and gender-appropriate growth charts. If a student had a BMI greater than or equal to 85% to 94% the diagnosis of overweight was made, and if their BMI was equal to or greater than 95% the diagnosis of obesity was made.[52]

Data analysis
Using correlation and regression analyses, relations among study variables were examined. Correlational analyses were used to examine the bivariate relations among intent to treat approach, a series of mixed-model analyses of variance examined the interaction between BMI and obesity and asthma QOL. Regression analyses were used to determine which variables predicted significant variability in asthma QOL. Finally, a series of *t*-tests were conducted to determine whether those who were overweight or obese had significantly worse outcomes than those who were of normal weight. Two-sided test were used and a *P* value of less than .05 was considered significant.

Results
At baseline, self-reported asthma QOL scores indicated a moderate level of impairment for all students, with only 53% of students determined to be in control of their asthma. Correlational results indicated that BMI was negatively associated with asthma QOL at baseline ($r = -0.16$), 2 months ($r = -0.10$), 6 months ($r = -0.09$), and 12 months ($r = -0.24$), although this relationship was only significant at 12 months ($P<.01$). These findings suggest that increased BMI is negatively associated with self-reported asthma QOL.

To further explore the nature of the relation between BMI and asthma QOL, *t*-tests were conducted to determine whether those who were overweight or obese had significantly worse asthma QOL relative to those who were of normal weight. Results indicated that those who were overweight or obese at baseline had marginally significantly lower asthma QOL (mean = 4.65, standard deviation [SD] = 1.11) compared with those who were normal weight (mean = 4.97, SD = 0.83), $t(121) = 1.78$, $P = .07$. Furthermore, at 12 months, those who were overweight or obese reported higher levels of negative coping (mean = 1.42, SD = 0.63) compared with those who were of normal weight (mean = 1.20, SD = 0.52), $t(121) = 2.06$, $P = .04$. In addition, those who were not in control of their asthma reported lower asthma QOL (mean = 4.67, SD = 1.10), $t(132) = 2.51$, $P = .01$. There were no significant differences between those who were overweight or obese and those who were normal at any other time point.

To examine the role of BMI in determining asthma QOL relative to other important predictors, a series of regression equations tested the relative importance of BMI in asthma QOL. Results indicated that when including symptom frequency, asthma classification (intermittent, mild, moderate, severe), asthma knowledge, asthma self-efficacy, and asthma self-care levels, BMI remained the strongest predictor of asthma QOL ($\beta = -0.28$, $P = .002$) along with asthma knowledge ($\beta = 0.28$, $P = .003$). These findings suggest that even when controlling for the influence of symptom frequency and asthma classification, BMI remains a most important factor in determining self-reported QOL among teens with asthma.

To determine whether BMI and obesity inhibits the effectiveness of an asthma treatment program (TEAM), an additional series or regression models were used to test the moderating role of BMI and obesity. Contrary to hypotheses, results indicated that when controlling for baseline levels of asthma QOL, neither BMI nor obesity had a significant moderating effect on the effectiveness of an asthma treatment program at 6 months ($\beta = -0.07$, $P = .82$; $\beta = 0.03$, $P = .86$, respectively). Similarly, when controlling for baseline levels of asthma QOL, neither BMI nor obesity had a significant moderating effect on the effectiveness of an asthma treatment program on asthma QOL at 12 months ($\beta = -0.05$, $P = .73$; $\beta = 0.03$, $P = .91$, respectively). These findings suggest that although BMI and obesity are important predictors of asthma-related QOL in their own right, they did not influence the effectiveness of the asthma treatment program in this study.

Discussion and Clinical Implications

Although the results showed that overweight and obesity did not change the effectiveness of the asthma treatment program, the impact obesity plays on QOL should not be ignored.

These findings support previous literature suggesting that overweight/obese adolescents experience poorer physical health than their nonoverweight peers. In a sample of 923 adolescents, Wake and colleagues[53] found that obesity was associated with a lower QOL. However, special needs related to asthma only slightly rose with increased BMI, and not to the point of significance. It was found that many adverse health and psychological effects of childhood obesity could be reversed if the obesity were treated before adolescence. However, specific health problems that would prompt a reduction in the BMI of adolescence were not reported. Although the strength of the random sampling method, parallel adolescent self-reports and parent proxy reporting, and large sample size add weight to the study findings, the study was limited by potential bias owing to attrition and a higher rate of obese participants lost.

In another study, Burkhart and colleagues[18] found that gender was statistically significantly associated with QOL in a sample of 30 adolescents with asthma. Males had a higher QOL compared with females ($P = .003$), and QOL scores were poorer with the experience of an asthma attack in the past 6 months. Asthma severity did not correlate with asthma QOL. However, the majority of the participants reported their asthma as mild (57%) and more than half said their activity was occasionally limited by asthma (56%). This study lends interesting insights into the predictors of QOL in adolescents with asthma; however, the weight of the contribution is limited by the small sample size, exploratory nature, and cross-sectional design.

The literature to date does highlight existing gaps and provides several outlets for future research. The comorbid prevalence of obesity and asthma in youth is clearly an area requiring to be understood. It is evident that health disparities exist for both asthma and obesity, especially in both Hispanic and African American youth. It is suggested that for these at-risk populations, weight-management and weight-reduction education should be included in every health-related visit. In addition, because of the negative effect of asthma and obesity on QOL, tools such as the Pediatric AQLQ should be used at every asthma evaluation visit, and QOL issues discussed as well as being incorporated into the asthma treatment plan.

REFERENCES

1. Flegal KM, Carroll MD, Kit BK, et al. Prevalence of obesity and trends in the distribution of body mass index among US adults, 1999-2010. JAMA 2012;307(5): 491–7.
2. Ogden CL, Carroll MD, Kit BK, et al. Prevalence of obesity and trends in body mass index among US children and adolescents, 1999-2010. JAMA 2012; 307(5):483–90.
3. Ford ES, Mannino DM. Time trends in obesity among adults with asthma in the United States: findings from three national surveys. J Asthma 2005;42(2): 91–5.
4. Chen AY, Kim SE, Houtrow AJ, et al. Prevalence of obesity among children with chronic conditions. Obesity 2009;17(6):1–4.
5. Akerman MJ, Calacanis CM, Madsen MK. Relationship between asthma severity and obesity. J Asthma 2004;41(5):521–6.
6. Luder E, Ehrlich RI, Lou WY, et al. Body mass index and the risk of asthma in adults. Respir Med 2004;98(1):29–37.
7. Spivak H, Hewitt MF, Onn A, et al. Weight loss and improvement of obesity-related illness in 500 U.S. patients following laparoscopic adjustable gastric banding. Am J Surg 2005;189(1):27–32.
8. Gennuso J, Epstein LH, Paluch RA, et al. The relationship between asthma and obesity in urban minority children and adolescents. Arch Pediatr Adolesc Med 1998;152:1197–2000.
9. Belamarich PF, Luder E, Kattan M, et al. Do obese inner-city children with asthma have more symptoms than nonobese children with asthma? Pediatrics 2000; 106(6):1436–41.
10. Rodriguez MA, Winkleby MA, Ahn D, et al. Identification of population subgroups of children and adolescents with high asthma prevalence: findings from the Third National Health and Nutrition Examination Survey. Arch Pediatr Adolesc Med 2005;156(3):269–75.
11. Visness CM, London SJ, Daniels JL, et al. Association of childhood obesity with atopic and non-atopic asthma: results from the National Health and Nutrition Examination Survey 1999-2006. J Asthma 2010;47:822–9.
12. Black MH, Smith N, Porter AH, et al. Higher prevalence of obesity among children with asthma. Obesity 2012;20:1041–7.
13. Chu YT, Chen WY, Wang TN, et al. Extreme BMI predicts higher asthma prevalence and is associated with lung function impairment in school-aged children. Pediatr Pulmonol 2009;44(5):472–9.
14. Sithole F, Douwes J, Burstyn I, et al. Body mass index and childhood asthma: a linear association? J Asthma 2008;45(6):473–7.
15. Noal RB, Menezes AMB, Macedo EC, et al. Childhood body mass index and risk of asthma in adolescence: a systematic review. Obes Rev 2011;12:93–104.
16. Mannino DM, Mott J, Ferdinands J, et al. Boys with high body masses have an increased risk of developing asthma: findings from the National Longitudinal Survey of Youth (NLSY). Int J Obes 2006;30:6–13.
17. Centers for Disease Control and DC. Healthy People. 2020. Available at: www. cdc.gov/nchs/healthy-people.htm. Accessed July 20, 2012.

18. Burkhart P, Svavardottir EK, Rayens MK, et al. Adolescents with asthma: predictors of quality of life. J Adv Nurs 2009;64(4):860–6.
19. Velsor-Friedrich B, Vlasses F, Moberley J, et al. Talking with teens about asthma management. J Sch Nurs 2004;20(3):140–8.
20. Bruzzese JM, Stepney C, Fiorino EK, et al. Asthma self-management is suboptimal in urban Hispanic and African American/black early adolescents with uncontrolled persistent asthma. J Asthma 2011;183:998–1006.
21. Everhart RS, Fiese BH. Asthma severity and child quality of life in pediatric asthma: a systematic review. Patient Educ Couns 2008;75:162–8.
22. Van De Ven MO, Engels RC, Sawyer SM, et al. The role of coping strategies in quality of life adolescents with asthma. Qual Life Res 2007;16:625–34.
23. Mohangoo AD, deKoning HJ, Mangunkusumg RT, et al. Health-related quality of life in adolescents with wheezing attacks. J Adolesc Health 2007;41(5): 464–71.
24. Schmier JK, Manjunath R, Halpern MT, et al. The impact of inadequately controlled asthma in urban children on quality of life and productivity. Ann Allergy Asthma Immunol 2007;98(3):245–51.
25. Bruzzese JM, Sheares BJ, Vincent JE, et al. Effects of a school-based intervention for urban adolescents with asthma. Am J Respir Crit Care Med 2011;49(1): 90–7.
26. Riekert KA, Borrelli B, Bilderback A, et al. The development of a motivational interviewing intervention to promote medication adherence among inner-city, African American adolescents with asthma. Patient Educ Couns 2011;82(1): 117–22.
27. Lavoie KL, Bacon SL, Labrecque M, et al. Higher BMI is associated with worse asthma control and quality of life but not asthma severity. Respir Med 2006; 100:648–57.
28. Grammer LC, Weiss KB, Pedicano JB, et al. Obesity and asthma morbidity in a community-based adult cohort in a large urban area: The Chicago Initiative to Raise Asthma Health Equity (CHIRAH). J Asthma 2010;47:491–5.
29. Peters JI, McKinney JM, Smith B, et al. Impact of obesity in asthma: evidence from a large prospective disease management study. Ann Allergy Asthma Immunol 2011;106:30–5.
30. Ravens-Sieberer U, Redegeld M, Bullinger M. Quality of life after in-patient rehabilitation in children with obesity. Int J Obes Relat Metab Disord 2001;25(S1): S63–5.
31. Blandon VV, del Rio Navarro B, Berber Eslava A, et al. Quality of life in pediatric patients with asthma with or without obesity: a pilot study. Allergol Immunopathol (Madr) 2004;32(5):259–64.
32. van Gent R, van der Ent CK, Rovers MM, et al. Excessive body weight is associated with additional loss of quality of life in children with asthma. J Allergy Clin Immunol 2007;119:591–6.
33. Michelson PH, Williams LW, Benjamin DK, et al. Obesity, inflammation, and asthma severity in childhood: data from the National Health and Nutrition Examination Survey 2001-2004. Ann Allergy Asthma Immunol 2009;103(5):381–5.
34. Coffman JM, Cabana MD, Yelin EH. Do school-based asthma education programs improve self-management and health outcomes? Pediatrics 2009; 124:729–42, 729.
35. Cristensin H, Griffins K, Korten A. Web-based cognitive behavior therapy: analysis of site usage and changes in depression and anxiety scores. J Med Internet Res 2002;4(1):e3.

36. Wright J. Cognitive behavior therapy. Basic principles and recent advances. Focus: The Journal of Lifelong Learning in Psychiatry American Psychology Association 2006;4(2):173–8.

37. Glick B. Cognitive behavioral interventions for at-risk youth. Kingston (NJ): Civic Research Institute; 2006.

38. Forman S. Coping skills for children and adolescents. San Francisco (CA): Josey-Bass; 1993.

39. Forman S, Linney J, Brondion M. Effects of coping-skills training on adolescents at risk for substance abuse. Psychol Addict Behav 1990;4:67–76.

40. Prinz R, Blechman E, Dumas J. An evaluation of peer coping-skills training for childhood aggression. Clin Child Fam Psychol Rev 1994;23:193–203.

41. Elias MJ, Gara M, Ubriaco M, et al. Impact of a preventive social problem solving intervention children's coping with middle-school stressors. Am J Community Psychol 1986;14:259–75.

42. Grey M, Boland E, Davidson M, et al. Coping skills training for youths with diabetes on intensive therapy. Appl Nurs Res 1999;12:3–12.

43. Grey M, Whittemore R, Jaser S, et al. Efforts of coping skills training in school-age children with type 1 diabetes. Res Nurs Health 2009;32:405–18.

44. Varni JW, Katz ER, Colegrove R, et al. The impact of social skills training on the adjustment of children with newly diagnosed cancer. J Pediatr Psychol 1993;18:751–67.

45. Jefferson V, Jaser S, Lindemann E, et al. Coping skills training in a telephone health coaching program for youth at risk for type 2 diabetes. J Pediatr Health Care 2011;25:153–61.

46. Grey M, Berry D, Davidson M, et al. Preliminary testing of a program to prevent type 2 diabetes among high-risk youth. J Sch Health 2004;74:10–5.

47. Velsor-Friedrich B, Militello L, Richards M, et al. Effects of coping skills training in low-income urban African-American adolescents with asthma. J Asthma 2011;49(4):372–9.

48. Junniper E, Guyatt G, Feeny D, et al. Measuring quality of life in children with asthma. Qual Life Res 1996;5:35–46.

49. Spirito A, Star L, Willimas C. Development of a brief coping checklist for use with pediatric populations. J Pediatr Psychol 1988;13:555–74.

50. Spirito A, Stark L, Kanpp L. Stress and coping in child health. In: Wallander JL, Walker CE, editors. The assessment of coping in chronically ill children: implications for clinical practice. New York: Guilford Press; 1992. p. 327–44.

51. National Asthma Education and Prevention Program. Expert Panel report. Guidelines for the diagnosis and management of asthma update on selected topics. 2007. Available at: http://www.nhlbi.nih.gov/guidelines/asthma/asthgdln.pdf. Accessed July 20, 2012.

52. Centers for Disease Control and Prevention (CDC). About BMI for children and teens. Available at: http://www.cdc.gov/healthyweight/assessing/bmi/childrens_bmi/about_childrens_bmi.html. Accessed May 27, 2012.

53. Wake M, Canterford L, Patton GC, et al. Comorbidities of overweight/obesity experienced in adolescence: longitudinal study. Arch Dis Child 2010;95:162–8.

Developing an Interactive Story for Children with Asthma

Tami H. Wyatt, PhD, RN[a],*, Xueping Li, PhD[b,c], Yu Huang, MS[d],
Rachel Farmer, MS, RN[e], Delanna Reed, PhD[f],
Patricia V. Burkhart, PhD, RN[g]

KEYWORDS

- Interactive story • Childhood asthma • Asthma management
- Internet based program • Asthma in school • Coping with asthma

KEY POINTS

- Interactivity is key to engaging school-aged children in asthma-management programs.
- School-aged children learn in story formats; hence, story is an appropriate teaching strategy for health-education programs for children.
- School-aged children can manage their own asthma if they are confident in their abilities and they have support of their peers, family, community, and health care team.
- Asthma programs for children should include ways to avoid asthma triggers; engage friends, families, school staff, and coaches; and teach strategies, such as monitoring lung function, stress reduction, and ways to cope with having asthma.

BACKGROUND AND SIGNIFICANCE

Asthma, an obstructive airway disease characterized by recurrent episodes of breathlessness and wheezing, is the most prevalent chronic illness among children in the United States.[1] Minority and low socioeconomic status patients are the most likely to be hospitalized for asthma.[2] The impact of this disease is striking: not only is asthma

Drs Wyatt & Li, National Institutes of Health, National Institute of Nursing Research 5R03NR011352.

[a] Educational Technology & Simulation, Health Information Technology & Simulation Lab, College of Nursing, University of Tennessee, 1200 Volunteer Boulevard, Knoxville, TN 37996, USA; [b] Ideation Laboratory, Department of Industrial and Systems Engineering, College of Engineering, University of Tennessee, 408 East Stadium Hall, Knoxville, TN 37996, USA; [c] Health Information Technology & Simulation Lab, Department of Industrial and Systems Engineering, College of Engineering, University of Tennessee, 408 East Stadium Hall, Knoxville, TN 37996, USA; [d] Department of Industrial and Systems Engineering, University of Tennessee, College of Engineering, 408 East Stadium Hall, Knoxville, TN 37996, USA; [e] Minute Clinic, 9137 Middlebrook Pike, Knoxville, TN 37931, USA; [f] Storytelling Program, East Tennessee State University, PO Box 70684, Johnson City, TN 37614, USA; [g] 202 College of Nursing, University of Kentucky, Lexington, KY 40536-0232, USA
* Corresponding author.
E-mail address: twyatt@utk.edu

the number 1 cause of hospitalizations for children aged 3 to 12, it also results in a total of 10.5 million missed school days per year.[3]

The tragedy is that many of these hospitalizations and missed school days are preventable. Better asthma management could save millions of dollars per year and spare patients with asthma and their families the trauma of a hospital stay.[4] Because children spend a significant amount time at school, it is important that they engage in self-care activities and seek help with self-management during these hours.

DEVELOPMENT OF AN INTERACTIVE ASTHMA PROGRAM

Okay with Asthma (OKWA) is a program for school-aged children that was designed for the school environment but may be well suited for home or clinic use.

Biobehavioral Family Model

OKWA uses the Biobehavioral Family Model (BBFM)[5] as a framework for the content, and therefore, promotes self-management skills with the help of family, peers, community, and health care providers. It also focuses on the importance of psychological and emotional functioning, including acceptance of asthma. Although OKWA will experience ongoing revisions owing to the nature of Internet sites, here we report the results of feasibility and usability testing with children as users of the program during focus groups.

It is clear that asthma management should include more than just information about medications and their uses. Asthma management includes identifying symptoms, reducing triggers that cause asthma, monitoring lung function, and knowing when and how to get help from others. In the BBFM, Wood and Miller[5] propose 3 overlapping "realms of functioning" that help determine the course of chronic childhood diseases: psychological and emotional functioning, social functioning (including family, school, peers, work), and biologic functioning (including the actual disease process). When these areas are balanced, the patient experiences a state of well-being. This state is interrupted if there is dysfunction in any of the realms. To keep balance, the child must draw on all available resources, including the family, health care providers, community, and peers.[5]

Studies have demonstrated the importance of the family in managing chronic conditions.[6] Encouraging strong family functioning can reduce child stress and improve asthma control.[6] Like other chronic conditions, asthma carries a strong psychosomatic component. Increased levels of child stress are correlated with increased asthma severity[7–9] and, therefore, may be considered an asthma trigger.

A child with well-managed asthma must feel secure in family relationships and know the family is reliable for problem solving.[7] Thus, an asthma education program using the BBFM would encourage a child to consider family members as resources to aid self-management; however, according to the BBFM, the family must not be the sole resource for managing chronic illness.[5] Dysfunctional families, or even families with limited financial means or a mother working outside the home, often have difficulty managing asthma,[10] and sometimes caregivers do not model effective coping strategies.

Keeping in mind that children spend most of their waking hours in school or school-related activities, the BBFM suggests that teaching children to seek resources at school could be empowering and helpful in managing asthma.[5] Existing literature supports school-based interventions, showing that they can help increase knowledge[11] and self-management.[12] Many children report concern about having an asthma attack at school and need encouragement to seek help from providers there.[13] Some research, however, shows programs with the greatest benefit involved advanced providers. Children who demonstrated fewer school absences during and after a school intervention program were those who met with an allergist and received a plan for asthma management.[12]

Hand-in-hand with the health care resources, the BBFM encourages accessing community resources. One study showed that home visits by a trained community health worker improved quality of life and reduced symptomatic days for patients in the Seattle area.[14]

Last, the BBFM proposes that peers be viewed as a resource for maintaining self-management of chronic diseases. In fact, evidence shows that children may rely on peers as an important part of their self-management. Peer acceptance, independent of asthma-related support, is correlated with healthy asthma lifestyle choices.[15] In the same study, it was found that parental support was only slightly more influential than peer support on asthma-related behaviors, such as managing asthma flares, avoiding causative substances, and maintaining a healthy level of physical activity. Educational initiatives led by peers can have an especially significant impact on attitudes and perception of quality of life, particularly in boys who have fewer family resources.[16]

All 4 factors outlined in the BBFM (family, health care, community, and peers) are significant in the management of chronic diseases like asthma. Researchers and providers would benefit from using this model to create educational materials that address not just one, but all of the factors, including the psychosocial strategies that are hallmark concepts of the BBFM.[7–9] One way to encourage children to manage their own asthma is to offer a BBFM-based educational program they can use at school.

Computer-Based Learning

Systematic reviews have repeatedly shown that interactive health communication applications positively affect knowledge, attitudes, behavior, and clinical outcomes.[17–19] Studies also indicate that computer-based learning (CBL) is especially helpful for elementary school students, as programs can help improve knowledge and attitudes[20] and increase problem-solving skills.[21] Interactive games also have shown great promise, both in increasing knowledge and improving clinical outcomes. An interactive game developed to improve asthma control among children aged 7 to 17 entitled "Watch, Discover, Think, and Act" was shown to increase self-efficacy, knowledge, and internal attributions.[22] Another study showed that low-income children who used the program had fewer asthma-related hospitalizations than their counterparts in the comparison group.[23] They also reported fewer asthma symptoms, less activity restriction, and better self-management behaviors than participants in the control group.[23]

OKWA

OKWA is an Internet-based program (www.okay-with-asthma.org), developed in 2003, that uses interactive narrative to teach asthma management to children aged 8 to 11. This award-winning program encourages users to describe their feelings and asthma support systems as they interact with a prewritten narrative and then add text to create their own stories. Because of the successes of the first version of OKWA, the developers planned a second version that uses similar, but more refined techniques supporting interactivity. The aim of this study was to test OKWAv.2.0's feasibility and usability (design, interactivity, functionality, and interface) during the development process by using focus groups with 8-year-old to 11-year-old children with asthma.

SELF-MANAGEMENT

The 2 main foci in developing OKWAv.2.0 were the program's content and delivery method. For the program to be most effective, its content must provide asthma self-management strategies that address all aspects (biopsychosocial) of the disease. In asthma, as in other chronic conditions, emphasis is placed on the concept of self-management. Children are urged to follow daily maintenance recommendations, perform regular monitoring, and appropriately treat acute and severe exacerbations. A Cochrane review of educational interventions found that an increased emphasis on self-management was correlated with increased lung function and a greater perception of self-control of the condition. Self-management also decreased loss of productivity and reduced asthma-focused emergency room visits.[24] The key to increased self-management is education.[25,26] Some children and families are unable to manage the disease because they have little concept of their ability to do so,[26] but educational interventions can help empower patients and caregivers to take control. Although research has indicated that patient education by a health care provider is helpful, some studies are investigating the role trained laypeople play in asthma education. Horner and Faloudi[11] found that classroom instruction by a lay educator improved students' knowledge of skills and perceived self-efficacy related to asthma control.

TODAY'S SCHOOL-AGED LEARNERS

Another crucial component in the success of OKWAv.2.0 is its attention to the specific needs of today's learners. To engage children,[27] programs must adopt multimedia-rich delivery methods that entertain while educating, especially programs designed to promote healthy behaviors.[28] In addition to using a multimedia-rich delivery system, OKWAv.2.0 uses interactive narrative, another effective strategy for educating children.

Engagement is a term often used to describe a user's relationship with an educational medium, including CBL programs. For learning to take place, a user must be engaged with the material.[29] Engagement can be defined as the user having positive emotional responses while his or her complete interest is held by the program; this may or may not include becoming unaware of time and the presence of others.[30] One theoretical framework for constructing engaging materials is the Engaging Multimedia Design Model, now renamed the Norma Engaging Multimedia Design (NEMD).[31] In a study that examined children's interaction with the computer game "The Sims," Norma Said identified 5 factors that facilitated engagement: simulation interactivity, construct interactivity, immediacy, feedback, and goals.[31] Simulation interactivity describes the child's ability to "become" a character in the story, whereas construct interactivity refers to the availability of activities for the child to create or build in the virtual world. Immediacy is the user's ability to observe all the actions and interactions that take place in the system. Children need feedback to show that their choices matter; without consequences, there would be no point in performing the actions. The model's final tenet is goal setting. Whether the goal is set extrinsically (by the game developer) or intrinsically (the child determining own goals), it is important for there to be goals to achieve.[32] The NEMD is one of the models used to guide the usability and feasibility testing of OKWAv.2.0 in this study.

INTERACTIVE NARRATIVES

Narratives, or stories, are an essential component in oral history, passing of traditions, and presenting lessons for preschool and school-aged children. As technology advances, narrative continues to be an essential experience; even computer games rely on narrative to give meaning to virtual activities.[19] To be effective, narratives must have a consistent and coherent plot containing elements of drama as well as character believability and empathy. The narrative must provide some aspects the user can control, and should promote positive emotions for the duration of use. Interactive narrative (IN) is a nonlinear story that allows users to select information, scenes, and characters (interactive) while developing a sequence of events (narrative) that culminates in a lesson or event.[33–35]

Unlike traditional forms of story, IN encourages active learning because the learner manipulates the content and plot of the narrative based on their input.[36] Interactive narratives have the potential to meet a learner's needs and encourage expression of thought and feelings while creating one's own personal asthma narrative. Interactive narrative as an intervention has been successfully used to increase knowledge and decrease symptoms and emergency room visits in children with asthma.[37]

OKWAv.2.0 allows the user to construct multiple, nonlinear stories. In fact, it is a story tree where branches of the story are different but each story shares the same trunk of characters and lessons pertaining to asthma **Fig. 1**. The interactivity of the story tree is designed to engage learners using the methods presented in the NEMD.[31] Using this design model may capture and retain the attention of children better than previous asthma programs, giving them multiple opportunities to express their own experiences and potentially learn new information with each use. Because children will likely create stories that are based on their own illness narrative or one they desire, OKWAv.2.0 may give families and health care providers, including school nurses, information about a child's perceived illness they might not otherwise receive.[38]

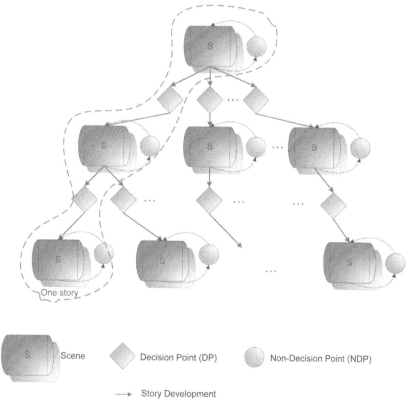

Fig. 1. OKWA v2.0 interactive narrative story tree.

BUILDING WITH CHILDREN

OKWAv.2.0 was built using an iterative process, which requires the user to evaluate and give feedback at intervals while the program is being developed. In this way, developers are interacting with users throughout the entire process of developing a program. This process, known as rapid prototyping,[39] is common in the software development industry but may not be as common while building applications for children because software testers are from the same demographic for which the program is being built. This requires children to participate in focus groups, which occurred in this usability study. Usability rules or heuritistics, developed by Jakob Nielsen, a nationally recognized expert in Web design and usability testing, guided the testing and analysis of content and functionality for OKWAv2.0. According to Nielsen,[40–42] Web-based applications are evaluated on 5 components: *learnability, efficiency, memorability, errors, and satisfaction.* Nielsen[40–42] also states that testing should occur by the same users who represent the population for which the application is designed. For this reason, children with asthma helped develop OKWAv2.0 and gave feedback and suggestions at intervals during the year that OKWAv.2.0 was developed.

SELECTING ASTHMA CONTENT AND NARRATIVES

To test the feasibility and usability of OKWA, the asthma content for OKWAv.2.0 was updated and reflects the National Asthma Education and Prevention Program, Panel 3.[42] The report was thoroughly examined and a list of key content was created to be included in each of the story branches. A childhood asthma expert who practices in a regional children's acute care hospital reviewed the asthma curriculum for accuracy and completeness.

Next, the research and development team created a list of activities, settings, and storylines that would appeal to children. Those children acquainted with the developers were informally polled and selected their 2 favorite story ideas. A storywriter incorporated the asthma content into 2 narratives: children snowboarding and children on a school playground. Because the storywriter was not a health care provider, it was necessary to consult with her frequently to explain content and ensure the asthma curriculum was incorporated appropriately. The 2 narratives served as a foundation or trunk for the story trees. The stories were broken into scenes. At various points in the 2 stories, a decision point was added so that a user could determine the sequence of the narrative based on their decision (refer to **Fig. 1**). The decision points created a total of 5 different stories, or branches, per story tree.

GRAPHICS AND FUNCTION OF OKWAV.2.0

A graphics artist created the scenes and characters, including character parts, such as arms and feet in various positions, to create the animation effects. The characters are ethnically and culturally diverse to represent communities across the United States. The same characters were used in both story trees and in all the branches of the story tree. Children who volunteered from local churches were audio recorded while reading lines from the stories, only after giving verbal consent, which was also recorded and is stored with the audio files. Once the stories came to life with characters, select scenes were drafted onto a Web page so that children in focus groups could begin evaluating components of OKWAv2.0. The program was built with Flash authoring software and can be viewed on all operating systems and browsers using the most current Flash player.

CONDUCTING FOCUS GROUPS
Methods and Procedures

After this the study was approved by the institutional review boards of the affiliated university and the local public school board, children with asthma between 8 and 11 years of age were recruited from primary schools in a metropolitan area in the southeastern region of the United States. The School Health Coordinator for the county helped identify schools in the inner city region with higher prevalence of asthma, and lower socioeconomic families based on the public school free-lunch program. Nurses at each school reviewed school records, identified potential participants, and then addressed and distributed a recruitment letter, which was sent home via the child. To ensure that confidential information about a child's health record was not revealed until after consent from a parent was obtained, the researchers were not privy to those families who received the recruitment letters. The recruitment letters, however, were returned to the researchers and included family contact information and the child's name. This process ensured the confidentiality of children whose families opted not to participate in this usability study. After parental or guardian consent and child assent were obtained, 6 focus groups were scheduled at 5 different schools. Some of the focus groups occurred during lunch, others occurred before the instructional day began or during the gym period. Scheduling was an important aspect of the process to ensure the study did not interrupt instructional time during the school day. The focus groups, lasting between 30 and 45 minutes, occurred in either the computer laboratory or the library at each school, with each child using a computer because the program is Internet based. Children were given headsets so that each child could work independently at his or her own pace. Children were neither given instructions about how to navigate the program nor were they given help while viewing unless they were unable to proceed. This technique is an important aspect in determining faulty navigation and functioning and to observe children exploring with the mouse. Children were encouraged to seek assistance if necessary and revisit scenes or sections as often as desired. During focus groups, a member of the research team made observations and field notes while children were quietly viewing the program and during the question-and-answer portion of the focus groups. The activities of each focus group varied, as well as the number of users, ages, and race. See **Table 1** for a description of the demographics for all focus groups.

Focus group 1 (FG1) evaluated the characters and 3 scenes from the snowboarding story and 2 scenes from the school playground story. The scenes had limited function and very few features, so the children could focus on the characters and the navigation structure from one scene to the next. Scenes with multiple characters were created with limited function. Children were instructed to begin the program from the home page and visit the pages as often as desired. Children were also instructed to remove their headset once they had previewed all pages. After all children completed this activity, they were asked to describe: (1) what they liked and disliked about the scenes, (2) their favorite character and why, (3) what they expected to happen next, (4) how they moved from one page to the next, (5) what they heard, (6) how they would go back to previous pages, and (7) what they learned about asthma.

Focus group 2 (FG2) evaluated 1 complete snowboarding story and 1 complete school playground story, which incorporated the feedback from FG1. Each story included interactive buttons that reinforced asthma content and gave trivia facts, such as famous persons with asthma. The 2 stories included voices for all characters, as well as animation in both stories. During FG2, children focused on the navigation to move from one scene to the next, active icons and links to learn more information, and how to change from one story branch to the other by answering the decision-point

Table 1
Total study demographics (all focus groups)

	FG 1	FG2	FG3	FG4	FG5	FG6	Total
Ethnicity							
Hispanic or Latino	1	–	–	–	–	2	3
Not Hispanic or Latino	8	1	3	6	9	3	30
Race							
American Indian	–	–	–	–	–	–	–
Alaska Native	–	–	–	–	–	–	–
Asian	–	–	–	–	–	–	–
Black	4	–	2	4	4	3	17
White	5	1	1	2	5	2	16
Age							
8	1	–	–	1	2	–	4
9	2	1	1	2	3	1	10
10	2	–	2	1	4	2	11
11	4	–	–	2	–	2	8
Sex/Gender							
Male	5	1	1	4	3	5	19
Female	4	–	2	2	6	–	14
Setting							
Library	–	–	√	–	–	–	
Computer laboratory	√	√	–	√	√	√	
					Total participants		33

Abbreviation: FG, focus group.

questions. Children were encouraged to explain how to (1) move from one page to the next, (2) make the story change, (3) get more information about asthma, and (4) make the characters talk. Finally, children were asked to explain what they liked or disliked and what they would change about the program.

Focus group 3 (FG3) and focus group 4 (FG4) were nearly identical in their purpose, only FG3 reviewed scenes, decision points, navigation, and functionality of portions of the snowboarding story tree, whereas FG4 reviewed portions of the school playground story tree. Both focus groups were designed to ascertain engagement and the 5 factors as identified by the NEMD. Sample focus group questions included the following: (1) Have you ever been in a situation like Jake in the story? (2) What buttons did you push and what did they do? (3) Tell me all of the different things you saw and learned about in the story. (4) What happened to Jake and what did his friends do?

Focus group 5 (FG5) and focus group 6 (FG6) were identical and incorporated the greatest number of design and functionality changes based on feedback from FG3 and FG4. FG6 was the same as FG5 because the developers wanted a broader audience to review the entire OKWAv2.0 program and make recommendations for improvements. Questions in FG5 and FG6 were broad, open-ended questions to encourage children to express any thoughts, ideas, and likes and dislikes about OKWAv2.0.

Data Analysis

Field notes taken during each focus group were entered into an evaluation tool at the end of the focus group, as the information guided each developmental stage of OKWAv2.0. Each item listed in the tool was evaluated by the research team to determine if it was a flaw in the program or merely a preference by the user. Those items deemed preferences were considered by the developers only if the preference appeared on multiple occasions, which never occurred. Those items deemed usability flaws were scored and ranked according to the importance of correcting the function and the feasibility of addressing the flaw. Those items ranking highest were addressed and changed in OKWAv2.0 before the next scheduled focus group. See **Table 2** for a sample evaluation tool.

Focus Group Study Results

In general, children engaged in the same activities while using OKWAv2.0. Many of the children looked over their shoulder or to the side to ensure their counterparts were experiencing the same scenes. Sometimes, the children in the focus groups would give or elicit help to their peers. Not surprising, the children appeared more comfortable relying on one another than asking the researchers for assistance. It can be assumed the children were more comfortable with one another than with the developers whom they had just met. The greatest revisions occurred between FG3–4 and FG5, in part, because FG3 and FG4 presented a complete IN with new features, icons, and buttons not seen previously. Based on user feedback, few changes were made to the storylines and scenes and no changes were made to the characters and their voices. The greatest changes occurred with the navigation and action buttons. A variety of buttons were used throughout the story pages so that users of the program could report their button preferences and researchers could observe user behavior while selecting buttons. Navigation and interactive buttons proved to be the greatest challenge for users. It was not obvious to the users whether to click on the speaker button to increase the volume or repeat what the character said. In some cases, the only way that children could identify a clickable object was by rolling the mouse over areas on the screen to reveal the "mickey mouse glove" or active link. Instructions and a key to the icons were added at the beginning of each story **Fig. 2**.

During FG3, an 11-year-old user grew frustrated because she could not start the story over before getting to the end of the story. The developers did not anticipate the need for this type of navigation, but as a result of this feedback, a link was added

Table 2
Sample evaluation tool of Okay with Asthma v2.0

Focus Group 1		Importance					Ease of Achievement					
Okay with Asthma v2.0 Content Issues	Preference or Flaw?	Low............High					Difficult............Easy					Product
		1	2	3	4	5	1	2	3	4	5	
I can't hear Jakes voice.	Flaw	☐	☐	☐	☐	☒	☐	☐	☒	☐	☐	15
Am I supposed to click on [nebulizer]?	Flaw	☐	☐	☐	☐	☒	☐	☐	☐	☒	☐	20
Do I click on [ear] to make the sound go up?	Flaw	☐	☐	☐	☐	☒	☐	☐	☐	☒	☐	20
I think those trees on the slope are too skinny.	Preference	☐	☐	☐	☒	☐	☐	☐	☐	☒	☐	16
What is an action plan?	Flaw	☐	☐	☒	☐	☐	☐	☐	☒	☐	☐	9

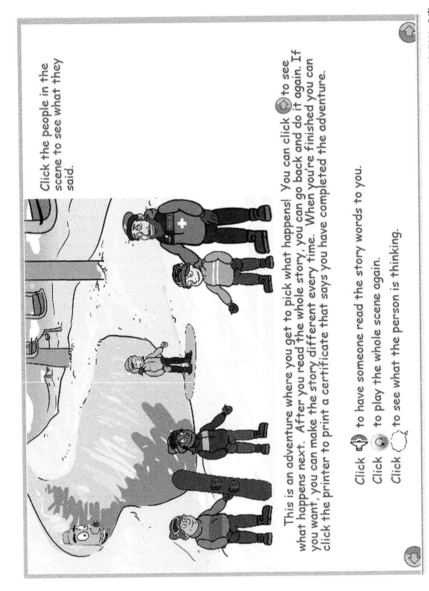

Click the people in the scene to see what they said.

This is an adventure where you get to pick what happens! You can click ⬆ to see what happens next. After you read the whole story, you can go back and do it again. If you want, you can make the story different every time. When you're finished you can click the printer to print a certificate that says you have completed the adventure.

Click 🎧 to have someone read the story words to you.

Click 🔄 to play the whole scene again.

Click 💭 to see what the person is thinking.

Fig. 2. Navigation instructions page. (*Courtesy of Okay with Asthma v2.0. Available at:* http://www.okay-with-asthma.org/OKWAv2/final/OKWA2.htm; with permission.)

App Name   **Okay With Asthma**

Description   **Okay with Asthma! is a website for school–aged children with asthma. Through an interactive story, children learn ways to manage and cope with their asthma. Okay with Asthma v2 is different from other from other asthma education programs about asthma because it focuses on the importance of school, friends and peers in managing asthma. Visit our site for more information at http://okay–with–asthma.org//.**

OKWA is an adventure where you get to pick what happens! You can click next to choose what happen next. After you read the whole story you can go back and do it again. If you want, you can make the story different every time.

Keywords   **Education, Child, Asthma**

Support Email Address   **iLab.utk@gmail.com**

Support URL   **http://okay–with–asthma.org//**

Marketing URL (Optional)

Privacy Policy URL
(Optional)

iPad Screenshots

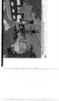
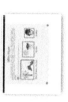

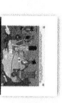
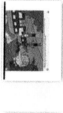
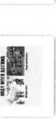

Fig. 3. Mobile application of OKWAv2.0.

so that a user could move to the previous page and start the story from the beginning at any scene in the story.

During one focus group, the users grew concerned that the main character asked for help from a stranger, which initiated a discussion about who should help someone with asthma. The users described ways they identified "safe" people, which was typically by their clothing. Mr Jim Hansen, the ski patrol in the snowboarding scene who helps the main character with asthma, was revised to include a red cross logo on his ski jacket along with a hat. In essence, the children helped to identify an important aspect of seeking help from others—identifying a trustworthy and safe person.

FUTURE VERSIONS OF OKWA

In many cases, users presented ideas that were not feasible to adopt in OKWAv2.0 because of budget constraints but these ideas will be considered in future versions. Some children in the focus groups wanted to pick a character representing themselves. Others wanted to create a character from parts like clothing articles, or hair and skin color. As expected, some children wanted active elements added to the story that had little or nothing to do with asthma or the plot of the story. For example, some users wanted all of the characters in the school playground story to sing a song and all of the boy characters in the snowboarding story to do somersaults on the slope.

An unexpected positive outcome occurred during FG6. Inner-city schools in a metropolitan area were targeted because of the relationship between asthma and children living in inner cities, but the school setting for the last focus group had a student body of mostly Hispanic population. In fact, the principal estimated that 80% of the students were Hispanic. Many of the teachers were bilingual in Spanish and English to communicate with the families of their pupils. Although the children were attending schools with English as the primary language, the parents or guardians were not English speaking, and, therefore, could not read English or the recruitment and consent letters prepared for this study. Spanish versions of the recruitment letter and the consent and assent forms were prepared and approved by the institutional review board. Two of the study participants in the last focus group were children of Spanish-speaking parents and required the Spanish version of the study forms, as well as an interpreter during the consent process. Future versions of OKWA will also include a Spanish version.

Not surprising, many of the children asked about a mobile application of the interactive narrative despite not owning a smart phone. Hence, a mobile version of OKWAv2.0 has already been created (**Fig. 3**). Children also inquired about additional stories and suggested stories that include swimming, playing instruments, and team sports, such as soccer or baseball.

SUMMARY

OKWAv.2.0 includes content from the latest guidelines of the National Asthma Education Prevention Program, Panel 3.[43] The program also allows children to interact with the characters and make decisions that influence the outcome of the story. This is an enhanced interactive feature that was not included in the first version. One aspect of the first version of OKWA that was lost in this version is the child's ability to add text to a comic strip story that could be printed. This feature will be considered if evaluations reveal that adding personal text and printing a story are essential to OKWA. Enhancements and revisions to OKWA resulted from feedback by children, specifically, children between 8 and 11 years of age with asthma. Obtaining evaluation data from children through focus groups is not common practice when designing health-related educational programs, but to dismiss children from participating in the evaluation and development of such programs is short sided. It is possible that programs built without children's input will be ill suited for them and appeal only to the adults who created the program.

Self-paced health-education programs, such as OKWAv2.0, are useful in a variety of settings provided the content is not facility specific. Children with asthma must learn to engage resources and assistance from others in a variety of places and settings, just as is presented in the BBFM.[5] OKWAv2.0 is intended for use in school clinics, but may be adopted for use in patient waiting rooms, hospital rooms, or at home. These programs, however, are only valued and visited frequently if the content is current, updated, and changes frequently or offers some function that invites the user to revisit the program again.

With technology advancements, it is now possible to make a story come alive in ways not possible before except through imagination, play, or with props, screen-writers, and sets. Now, stories can be interactive with multiple media, such as animation and sound, and they can change and evolve based on selections or decisions made by a user. In essence, interactive stories are the simplest forms of technology gaming but despite their simplicity, they are enticing for school-aged children. This might be because of the school-aged child's cognitive development and computer skills or it may be that children are enamored with stories: stories in story time at the library, storylines in plays, storylines in movies, and storylines in games.

Technology will continue to advance and the treatment of asthma will also improve. A wish list for future versions of OKWA is growing and includes more stories, the ability to build a character by selecting physical features or clothes, and stories in multiple languages. Additional story trees, new characters, and added interactive features will keep children visiting and learning how to seek help from others, avoid triggers, manage their asthma, and learn to live with their asthma.

REFERENCES

1. Egan K. The educated mind: how cognitive tools shape our understanding. Chicago: University of Chicago Press; 1997.
2. Asthma and Allergy Foundation of America. Asthma Capitals. The Asthma Capitols; annual report funded by AstraZeneca. Available at: http://aafa.org/pdfs/FinalPublicListAC2008.pdf. Accessed August 22, 2012.
3. Akinbami LJ, Moorman JE, Liu X. Asthma prevalence, health care use, and mortality: United States, 2005-2009. Natl Health Stat Report 2011;32:1–14.
4. Ordõnez GA, Phelan PD, Olinsky A, et al. Preventable factors in hospital admissions for asthma. Arch Dis Child 1998;78(2):143.
5. Wood BL, Miller BD. A biopsychosocial approach to child health. In: Kaslow FW, editor. Comprehensive handbook of psychotherapy. 4th edition. New York: John Wiley & Sons; 2002. p. 59–79.
6. Ng SM, Lou VW, Tso IF, et al. Incorporating family therapy into asthma group intervention: a randomized wait-list controlled trial. Fam Process 2008;47(1):115–30.
7. Wood BL, Lim J, Miller BD, et al. Testing the biobehavioral family model in pediatric asthma: pathway of effect. Fam Process 2008;47(1):21–40.
8. Wood BL, Klebba KB, Miller BD. Evolving the biobehavioral family model: the fit to attachment. Fam Process 2000;39(3):319–44.
9. Wood BL, Miller BD, Hungha L, et al. Family relational factors in pediatric depression and asthma: pathways of effect. J Am Acad Child Adolesc Psychiatry 2006; 45(12):1494–502.

10. Bloomberg GR, Banister C, Sterkel R, et al. Socioeconomic, family and pediatric practice factors that affect level so asthma control. Pediatrics 2009;123(3):829–35.
11. Horner SD, Fouladi RT. Improvement of rural children's asthma self-management by lay health educators. J Sch Health 2008;78(9):506–13.
12. Bartholomew LK, Parcel GS, Kok G, et al. Planning health promotions programs: an intervention mapping approach. San Francisco (CA): Jossey-Bass; 2006.
13. Meng A, McConnell S. Decision-making in children with asthma and their parents. J Am Acad Nurse Pract 2002;14(8):363–71.
14. Krieger J, Takaro TK, Song L, Beaudet N, et al. A randomized controlled trial of asthma self-management support comparing clinic-based nurses and in-home community health workers: the Seattle-King county healthy homes II project. Arch Pediatr Adolesc Med 2009;163(2):141–9.
15. Yang TY, Sylva K, Lunt I. Parent support, peer support and peer acceptance in healthy lifestyle for asthma management among early adolescents. J Spec Pediatr Nurs 2010;15:272–81.
16. Rhee H, Belyea MJ, Hunt JF, et al. Effects of a peer-led asthma self-management program for adolescents. Arch Pediatr Adolesc Med 2011;165(6):513–9.
17. Murray E, Burns J, See TS, et al. Interactive Health Communication Applications for people with chronic disease. Cochrane Database of Systematic Reviews 19(4);CD004274. Available at: http://www.ucl.ac.uk/slms/people/show.php?person id=12015.
18. Lieberman DA. Management of chronic pediatric diseases with interactive health games: theory and research findings. J Ambul Care Manage 2001; 24(1):26–38.
19. Baranowski T, Buday R, Thompson DI, et al. Playing for real: video games and stories for health-related behavior change. Am J Prev Med 2008;34(1):74–82.
20. Palmer S, Graham G, Elliot E. Effects of web-based health program on fifth grade children's physical activity knowledge, attitudes and behavior. Am J Health Edu 2005;36:86–94.
21. Serin O. The effects of the computer-based instruction on the achievement and problem solving skills of the science and technology students. Turk Online J Dist Educ 2011;10(1):183–201.
22. Shegog R, Bartholomew KL, Parcel GS, et al. Impact of a computer-assisted education program on factors related to asthma self-management behavior. J Am Med Inform Assoc 2001;8:49–61.
23. Bartholomew LK, Gold RS, Parcel GS, et al. Watch, discover, think and act: evaluation of computer-assisted instruction to improve asthma self-management in inner-city children. Patient Educ Couns 2000;39:39–42.
24. Wolf FM, Guevara FP, Grum CM, et al. Educational interventions for asthma in children. Cochrane Database Syst Rev 2003;(1):CD000326.
25. Pruitt B. Controlling asthma takes a combination of tools, including pulmonary function test and most recently, looking at biomarkers. 2011. Available at: http://www.rtmagazine.com/issues/articles/2011-01_04.asp. Accessed September 20, 2012.
26. Burkhart PV, Rayens MK. Self-concept and health locus of control: factors related to children's adherence to recommended asthma regimen. Pediatr Nurs 2005; 31(5):404–9.
27. Mayer RE. Multi-media learning. New York: Cambridge University Press; 2001.
28. Huss K, Winkelstein ML, Crosbie K, et al. Backpack adventures in asthma: interactive multimedia computer game piques children's interest in asthma. J Allergy Clin Immunol 2001;107:239.

29. Bandura A. Social foundations for thought and action. A social cognitive theory. J Soc Clin Psychol 1986;4:359–74.
30. O'Brien HL, Toms EG. What is user engagement? A conceptual framework for defining user engagement with technology. J Am Soc Inform Sci Tech 2008; 59(6):938–55.
31. Said NS. An engaging multimedia design model. Proceedings of the 2004 conference on interaction design and children: building a community. New York; ACM; 2004. p. 169–72. http://dx.doi.org/10.1145/1017833.1017873.
32. Said N, Rahman S, Yassin SF. Revisiting an engaging experience to identify metacognitive strategies towards developing a multimedia design model. Int Educ Inform Tech 2009;3:2, 115–25.
33. Douglas JY. The end of book or books without end? Ann Arbor (MI): The University of Michigan Press; 2004.
34. Nelson MJ, Mateas M, Roberts DL, et al. Declarative optimization-based drama management in interactive fiction. IEEE Comput Graph Appl 2006;26(3):32–41.
35. Szilas N. A computational model of an intelligent narrator for interactive narratives. Appl Artif Intell 2007;21:753–801.
36. Marsella SC, Johnson WL, LaBore CM. Interactive pedagogical drama for health interventions. Proceedings from the 11th International Conference on Artificial Intelligence in Education. Sydney, July 20–24, 2004.
37. Krishna S, Balas EA, Spencer DC, et al. Clinical trials of interactive computerized patient education: implications for family practice. J Fam Pract 1997;45(1):25–33.
38. Rich M, Taylor SA, Chalfen R. Illness as a social construct: understanding what asthma means to the patient to better treat the disease. J Qual Improv 2000; 26(5):244–53.
39. Smith MF. Software prototyping: adoption, practice and management. London: McGraw-Hill; 1991.
40. Nielsen J. Finding usability problems through heuristic evaluation. Proceeding of the SIGCHI conference on human factors in computing systems. Available at: http://portal.acm.org/citation.cfm?id=142834. Accessed September 18, 2012.
41. Kahn MJ, Prail A. Formal usability inspections. In: Nielsen J, Mack RL, editors. Usability Inspection Methods. New York: John Wiley & Sons; 1994. p. 141–72.
42. Nielsen J. How to conduct a heuristic evaluation. Available at: www.useit.com/papers/heuristic/heuristic_evaluation.html. Accessed May 30, 2012.
43. National Heart, Lung and Blood Institute [NHLBI]. Expert panel report 3 (EPR2): Guidelines for the diagnosis and management of asthma. Available at: www.nhlbi.nih.gov/guidelines/asthma/asthgdln.htm. Accessed October 18, 2007.

Therapeutic Conversations Intervention in Pediatrics
Are They of Benefit for Families of Children with Asthma?

Anna Olafia Sigurdardottir, MSc, RN[a,b,*],
Erla Kolbrun Svavarsdottir, PhD, RN[a,b], Mary Kay Rayens, PhD[c],
Sarah Adkins, MSc[d]

KEYWORDS

- Family system nursing • Nursing intervention • Family perceived support • Asthma
- Health-related quality of life

KEY POINTS

- It is encouraging for nurses in pediatric clinical settings to administer the short-term family therapeutic conversation intervention for families of children and adolescents with asthma.
- Mothers of children and teenagers with asthma are often the primary caregivers; therefore, it is valuable in clinical settings to know the positive impact of the short-term family therapeutic conversation intervention on the mothers' perception of perceive family support as well as on the children's perception of fewer problems with asthma treatment.

Funding/Sponsorships: This study was funded by grants from Research Fund of Ingibjorg R. Magnusdottir, the Research Fund at LUH and Scientific Fund of Icelandic Nurses Association.
Disclosure: The authors listed in this disclosure have identified no financial affiliations for themselves or their spouse/partner: Anna Olafia Sigurdardottir, PhD (student), RN, Clinical Nurse Specialist and Clinical Assistant Professor at Landspitali - The National University Hospital in Iceland; Erla Kolbrun Svavarsdottir, PhD, RN, Professor, School of Health Sciences, Faculty of Nursing, University of Iceland and Head of research and development of family nursing at Landspitali - The National University Hospital in Iceland; Mary Kay Rayens, PhD, Professor, College of Nursing and College of Public Health, University of Kentucky, Lexington, KY; Sarah Adkins, MS, Assistant Professor, College of Justice & Safety, Eastern Kentucky University, Richmond, KY.
[a] Landspitali - The National University Hospital in Iceland, Landspitali 21D Hringbraut, Reykjavik 101, Iceland; [b] Faculty of Nursing, School of Health Sciences, University of Iceland, Reykjavik, Iceland; [c] College of Nursing and College of Public Health, University of Kentucky, Lexington, KY, USA; [d] College of Justice and Safety, Eastern Kentucky University, Richmond, KY, USA
* Corresponding author. Landspitali University Hospital in Iceland Landspitali 21D Hringbraut, Reykjavik 101, Iceland.
E-mail address: annaosig@landspitali.is

INTRODUCTION

Worldwide, asthma is one of the most common chronic illnesses among children and teenagers and the prevalence continues to increase. In the United States, asthma affects 8% to 14% of children younger than 17 years[1,2]; which is a similar prevalence to Iceland and Sweden, affecting about 9% of Icelandic and Swedish school-age children.[3] Even although childhood asthma prevalence has increased over the last decade, asthma hospitalization has decreased; which has resulted in the expectation of a greater involvement by parents in asthma caregiving activities.[1,4] However, because of pediatric asthma symptoms, visits to the emergency department and to primary care settings have increased, which suggests a need for specific tailored interventions regarding asthma education and support for the families.[1,5,6]

Uncontrolled asthma can be a life-threatening situation; therefore, it is vital for parents to be well informed about how to manage asthma symptoms. Asthma symptoms can include wheezing, coughing, shortness of breath, and chest tightness.[2] Because of the effect asthma symptoms can have on children's quality of life (QOL), health care providers may need to focus on daily asthma management. However, researchers have shown that less than half of the parents of children with asthma have ever received asthma education.[7] The traditional way to support families in asthma management is to educate parents about asthma control and asthma triggers. Nevertheless, research results have indicated that most admissions to hospitals because of asthma attacks could have been prevented, if asthma medications had been taken regularly and if known asthma triggers had been avoided.[4,5]

Interventions need to be developed and tested to support families, reduce asthma severity, and improve asthma management and QOL for families of children and adolescents with asthma. However, little theory-based research has been carried out to assess the effectiveness of interventions for families of children or adolescents with asthma. The purpose of this theory-based quasiexperimental intervention study was to evaluate the effectiveness of a brief family therapeutic conversation intervention (FAM-TC) for families of children with asthma, with the intervention focused on perceived family support and health-related QOL. This intervention study was developed as a part of a knowledge translation project, the Landspitali University Hospital (LUH) Family Nursing Implementation Project (2007–2009), with a systematic plan to translate knowledge into clinical practice.

BACKGROUND
Family Nursing Interventions: Asthma-Related QOL

A growing emphasis within health care settings is on involving families in health care and assessing the outcomes resulting from this involvement. Therefore, there is a need for nurses who are offering evidence-based practice to be creative in their effort to develop and implement intervention to families. Researchers working on translating knowledge into clinical practice have made family nursing more visible and have reported the benefit of involving families in nursing care.[8–14] Nevertheless, there is a dearth of research focused on the benefit of involving families in theory-driven asthma intervention studies, in which the key outcomes are family-level variables such as support, QOL, and functioning.

Most of the research published on families of children or adolescents with asthma focuses on asthma symptoms, management, and medication or on asthma triggers. A meta-analysis[5] was conducted on the needs of parents and children to recognize asthma symptoms, control environmental triggers, follow complex medication regiments, and be aware of the role each health care provider provides in asthma care.

Thirty-seven randomized controlled trials were evaluated in this analysis involving children ranging from 2 to 17 years old. The main finding from the meta-analysis[5] was that families who were given the asthma education had reduced hospitalizations and emergency visits compared with the families who received usual care. Similarly, in a systematic review on 38 research studies involving 7843 children with asthma and their families,[6] it was concluded that an intervention centered on asthma education was associated with reduced risk of visits to the emergency department and hospital admission for families of children in the intervention groups compared with families of children in the control groups. More recently, in a school-based stress-management feasibility intervention study for 7-year-old to 12-year-old children with asthma focusing on psychological education, stress and emotions, problem-solving and coping skills, training, and relaxation[15]; the investigators found the intervention to be helpful for high-risk school-age children with asthma in that they were better at identifying early signs of asthma, applied asthma management skills at early stages, and their asthma symptoms were better controlled.

Inadequately controlled asthma has been found to have a significant negative impact on asthma QOL[16]; therefore, involving parents in asthma management of their children is important, but the child's developmental state and autonomy need to be taken into consideration. Burkhart and colleagues[17] found that controlling asthma symptoms among 7-year-old to 11-year-old children with asthma improved the children's QOL, but the asthma was better controlled when the children and their families followed recommended asthma treatment.[17] Similarly, assessing asthma care in schools needs to be considered when asthma management is evaluated. Svavarsdottir and colleagues[18] found in a study of an international school nurse asthma project on adolescents with asthma that communication challenges with parents and teachers and time constraints were the main barriers indicated by school nurses to asthma care in schools in Iceland (n = 17) and in the United States (n = 15).[18]

There is strong evidence in the literature that pediatric asthma can have a significant impact on health-related QOL (HRQOL). Therefore, the use of pediatric QOL measures has increased, in an effort to improve pediatric patients' well-being and health and to determine the value of health care services.[19–21] Varni and Limbers[20] proposed that to improve the quality of health care services, QOL outcomes in collaboration with a consumer-based health care outcomes approach need to be measured on a regular basis, both from the perspective of the children and their parents.[20] In an international study of asthma QOL among 30 families of adolescents with asthma in the United States (n = 15) and in Iceland (n = 15), who were receiving health care services at outpatient pediatric clinics, the parents in both countries were found to rate their children's QOL as poorer than the adolescents rated their own QOL. Further, although the parents and the teens generally agreed on the impact of the symptoms that affected QOL, they did not perceive in the same way what impact problems with asthma treatment, worrying, and communication had on asthma-related QOL. Relative to the teens' own ratings of their QOL, US parents tended to underrate their child's QOL, whereas parents from Iceland overrated it.[22]

Practice Framework of Family System Nursing: Theoretic Background

The theoretic background that guided the study was the Calgary Family Assessment (CFAM) and the Calgary Family Intervention Models (CFIM).[9] In the CFAM, the focus is on assessing 3 major categories, including the structural, developmental, and functional categories of family life. The focus of the CFIM is on changing cognitive, affective, or behavioral domains of family functioning. Wright and Leahey[9] developed a short-term intervention (the 15-minute [or less] family nursing intervention) to meet the needs of nurses who wanted to implement the theoretic foundation of the CFIM into clinical practice. The main components of the intervention are manners, compiling a family tree, in which a map of the family relational network is created (genogram and ecomap), asking therapeutic questions, and offering commendations.[9]

This short-term intervention has been used successfully by practitioners, educators, and researchers around the world who are working with families experiencing acute or chronic illnesses or injuries. Through the years, the focus of family nursing research has been on the benefit of family system nursing (FSN) intervention, with coding of qualitative narratives as the primary analysis strategy.[9,10] However, recently, we have increasingly seen the use of quantitative analysis within the context of a designed study when the goal is to test the effectiveness of a family-centered intervention.[8,23–25] Research on the usefulness of the 15-minute family interview has been reported in pediatric practice, by using quantitative[26–28] and qualitative[8,11,13,14,29] analysis.

LeGrow and Rossen[27] examined the application of FSN in a pediatric rehabilitation center, from both the parents' and the nurses' perspectives. After applying FSN in practice, the nurses focused more on the family, paying particular attention to their communication and interaction with families, and reported more positive professional practices and an increase in their own self-esteem. From the families' perspective, they perceived increased friendliness and frequency of communication with the nurses, greater consistency of nursing care, and enhancement of rapport with the nurses.[27] In another study, on the influence of a family intervention from the nurse's perspective in the context of pediatric hospital admissions,[28] the nurses perceived that an awareness of the key components of the 15-minute family interview had a positive impact on their ability to conduct family assessments and interventions.

Further, Svavarsdottir and colleagues[13] found in a short-term therapeutic conversation intervention focusing on cognitive and emotional support among 76 families of acute or chronically ill children that the parents in the experimental group (n = 41) reported significantly higher family support after the intervention compared with the parents in the control group (n = 35).[13] Also, Kamban and Svavarsdottir[29] studied in a quasiexperimental research design the benefits of a pediatric family nursing intervention, in which families of young children with respiratory syncytial virus were offered a short-term FAM-TC focusing on psychosocial support and education at a pediatric emergency department. Mothers who were in the experimental group (n = 21) and received the short-term intervention reported a significant increase on perceived family support compared with the mothers who were in the control group (n = 20), who had received treatment as usual.[29] Pediatric nurses in clinical practices are in a great position to assist parents by informing them about the child's illness and by providing them with an opportunity to talk about their concerns.

Hypotheses and Research Questions

Based on the review of the literature and the conceptual framework that guided the study, it was hypothesized that (1) parents (mother and father) who received the brief FAM-TC intervention would perceive significantly higher family support (both total scale and subscales) than the parents in the control group who received treatment as usual; and (2) parents who received the FAM-TC intervention and their children with asthma would report similar or significantly higher asthma QOL after the parents had received the FAM-TC intervention, compared with the parents in the control group who received treatment as usual.

The following research questions were asked: (1) what is the difference before the intervention for the experimental group on perceived family support (total scale and subscales) based on the parent's gender? (2) What are the differences in family support (total score) and the cognitive and the emotional support subscales as reported by the mothers in the experimental group over time? (3) What are the differences before the intervention in family support (total score) and the cognitive and the emotional support subscales, as reported by the fathers in the experimental and the control groups? (4) What are the differences for the experimental group in the children's and the parents' asthma QOL scores?

METHODS
Design and Procedures

The study is a quasiexperimental intervention study, with a pretest and posttest study design. The families were introduced to the study by a clinical nurse specialist at the hospital, who invited eligible parents to participate. The inclusion criterion for the study was that children and adolescents had to be between 5 and 18 years of age and have at least 1 parent willing to participate in the study. The children had to have been diagnosed with asthma (*International Classification of Diseases, Tenth Revision* J45.9 and J46) at least 6 months before recruitment and were receiving health care related to asthma symptoms at LUH Children's Hospital for at least 1 year. The families also needed to be able to read and write Icelandic. Parents and the children were excluded if they were being treated for other major physical or mental health problems besides asthma. Written consent was obtained from both parents. The parents were assigned by convenience to either an experimental group or to a control group. All participants in both groups answered Web-based questionnaires (outcome survey) before and after the intervention; the postintervention survey was 10 to 14 days later after the second therapeutic conversation interview. Data were collected from both the parents and the children between May and September 2009.

The Brief FAM-TC Intervention

The brief therapeutic conversation intervention offered by the nurses to families of children and adolescents with asthma consists of 2 sessions of therapeutic conversation built on the conceptual framework of the CFIM (**Boxes 1** and **2**).[9] In the intervention, the main focus was on the assessment and on the key elements of the 15-minute-or-less family interview. The brief therapeutic conversation intervention was introduced to the parents as an opportunity for them to engage in a therapeutic

---

Box 1
The first session of the FAM-TC intervention

- The nurse introduced herself to the parents and stated the purpose of the study.

- The nurse in cooperation with the parents drew a genogram and an ecomap of the family, with a specific focus on identifying the quality of the parent's relationships with other family members, schools, friends, and the social support/institutions in the society.

- The nurse offered the parents some informative information regarding their child's health condition and asked therapeutic questions regarding the family's challenges because of the asthma situation and impact of the asthma situation on family members, and so forth.

- Specific questions were asked based on the child's asthma condition and on how the family was managing the asthma.

- The parents described their experiences of having their child diagnosed with asthma and responses from friends, teachers, schools, and health care professionals.

- At the end of the interview the nurse commended the families.

Box 2
The second session of the FAM-TC intervention

- The nurse asked if the parents had any specific questions from the last session.

- While the nurse and the family were having the therapeutic conversation, the nurse used the genogram and the ecomap from the last session to refer to family members, friends, work and school settings, and so forth.

- The nurse asked specific therapeutic questions related to siblings in the family, future expectation of the family regarding the asthma situation, and encouraged the parents to share their illness experiences and their illness narratives as well as to indicate their constraining and facilitating beliefs.

- Questions were asked based on the child's health condition.

- The parents were given time to reflect on their own experiences and express how they were dealing with the situation.

- When the interview had come to an end, the nurse thanked the parents for their participation and emphasized that they could always contact the research team if they had any questions regarding the interview and that they could also talk to the asthma team at the Children's Hospital.

---

relationship. Each family received 2 therapeutic conversation interviews, ranged from 45 to 90 minutes, averaging 60 minutes. After the parents had signed the consent form, and answered the Web-based questionnaires, the nurse accompanied the parents to the intervention room.

For all of the families who participated in the intervention, the second session was offered 10 to 14 days after the first session.

Procedure for Data Collection

Parents were invited to participate in this therapeutic conversation intervention by a clinical nurse specialist. The parents were assigned either to the experimental group, who received the 2-session FAM-TC intervention, or to the control group, who received the usual treatment that was offered to all families at that time. The data were collected by 2 nurses, who had received education and training on supervision in FSN. One had an MS degree in nursing with a special focus on FSN and the other nurse had worked at an outpatient clinic for children and adolescents with asthma for more than 10 years. The nurses were specially trained in offering and administering the FAM-TC intervention.

Sample

Sixteen families were offered participation in the experimental group, but 1 family declined, so 15 parents (94%) finished the study. In the control group, 18 families were introduced to the study, but 2 declined, so 89% of the parents who were approached completed the study. Data were then collected from these 31 families of children with asthma (31 mothers, 15 fathers, and 31 children with asthma) who were receiving health care service in 2009 at an outpatient clinic at the LUH Children's Hospital (**Table 1**).

Measurements

To evaluate the effectiveness of the interventions, 2 questionnaires were used for the mothers and the fathers: the ICE-Family Perceived Support Questionnaire (ICE-FPSQ) (Svavarsdottir EK, Sveinbjarnardottir EK. The ICE-Family Perceived Support Questionnaire. Unpublished manuscript. Reykjavik [Iceland]: University of Iceland,

Table 1

Demographic characteristics of families of children and adolescents with asthma who received the therapeutic conversation intervention (N = 31 families; n = 31 mothers; n = 15 fathers, n = 31 children)

Demographic Variable	Experimental Group		Control Group		Test Statistic	
	n	%	n	%	χ^2	P value
Child's gender						
Female	9	60.0	4	25.0	3.89	.05
Male	6	40.0	12	75.0		
Child's age (y)						
5–7	1	6.7	4	25.0	2.02	.4
8–12	5	33.3	5	31.2		
13–18	9	60.0	7	43.8		
Parental participation						
Mother only	8	53.3	8	50.0	0.03	.9
Both parents	7	46.7	8	50.0		
Age of mothers (y)						
19–30	0	0.0	2	12.4	4.05	.3
31–40	6	40.0	7	43.8		
41–50	7	46.7	7	43.8		
51–60	2	13.3	0	0.0		
Age of fathers (y)						
19–30	0	0.0	1	12.5	2.14	.5
31–40	4	57.1	4	50.0		
41–50	3	42.9	2	25.0		
51–60	0	0.0	1	12.5		
Marital status						
Married/cohabitating	13	86.7	12	75.0	0.68	.4
Divorced/single	2	13.3	4	25.0		
Mother's education						
Less than high school	0	0.0	0	0.0	0.54	.5
High school	6	42.9	9	56.3		
University	8	57.1	7	43.7		
Father's education						
Less than high school	0	0.0	0	0.0	0.03	.9
High school	5	71.4	4	66.7		
University	2	28.6	2	33.3		
Family income (Icelandic kroners per month, in thousands)						
<201–400	5	33.3	6	40.0	0.17	.9
401–600	3	20.0	3	20.0		
>601	7	46.7	6	40.0		

Faculty of Nursing; 2009) and the HRQOL (PedsQL Asthma module).[30] In addition, the parents answered information about the demographic status of the families, as well as the health condition of the child (Svavarsdottir EK, Sigurdardottir AO. Demographic information and characteristics of the child's health. Unpublished manuscript. Reykjavik [Iceland]: University of Iceland, Faculty of Nursing; 2009 and Svavarsdottir EK, Sigurdardottir AO. Asthma factor index questionnaire. Unpublished manuscript. Reykjavik [Iceland]: University of Iceland, Faculty of Nursing; 2009.) Then the children with asthma answered the PedsQL Asthma module questionnaire.

The demographic information included questions about the parents' age, marital status, education, family income, and so forth. Information regarding the children's health was collected by the 21-item Asthma factor index questionnaire. (Svavarsdottir EK, Sigurdardottir AO. Asthma factor index questionnaire. Unpublished manuscript. Reykjavik [Iceland]: University of Iceland, Faculty of Nursing; 2009.) In this questionnaire, data were collected regarding the child's asthma condition, such as the asthma medication, severity of the asthma, hospitalization, and support.

ICE-FPSQ is a 14-item instrument with 2 factors: cognitive support and emotional support. This questionnaire is a Likert-type scale, with a scoring procedure from 1 (almost never) to 5 (almost always). A higher score indicates a better perception of family support. The Cronbach α for the whole instrument has been reported to be 0.953, with $\alpha = 0.874$ for the cognitive subscale and $\alpha = 0.937$ for the emotional subscale.[31] The questionnaire was developed from the conceptual framework of CFIM. The Icelandic version of this instrument has been psychometrically tested and found to be both valid and reliable.[31]

HRQOL (PedsQL 3.0 Asthma module) was measured both from the parents' (mother and father), children's, and adolescents' perspective. Children and adolescents (5–18 years) responded to the original version and parents completed the children's and adolescents proxy report of this same instrument to rate their perceptions. The instrument has 28 items, with 5-point Likert-type responses, ranging from "never a problem" to "almost always a problem." Items are reverse-scored and rescaled to range from 0 to 100, with higher scores indicating a better QOL. The PedsQL 3.0 Asthma module comprises 4 subscales, all identifying a problem within the last month, including (1) asthma (11 items), (2) treatment problems (11 items), worrying (3 items), and communication (3 items). The PedsQL Asthma module has been found to be both valid and reliable, with the average Cronbach α of 0.860.[30] In this study of families of children with asthma, the Cronbach α for the parents ranged from 0.883 to 0.908 and for the children, $\alpha = 0.864$ to 0.963 over time.

Data Analysis

Descriptive analyses, including means and standard deviations or frequency distributions, were used to summarize the demographic characteristics, illness and environmental variables, and outcome variables at baseline and after intervention. Comparisons of the 2 intervention groups at baseline were accomplished with the χ^2 test of association, Fisher exact test or the 2-sample t test, as appropriate.

Repeated measures analysis of variance was used to assess intervention effects over time on the outcomes, including both the main effect and interaction effects. This series of models contained 2 within factors (time, with values of baseline and after intervention; family member, with values of mother, father, and child for QOL total and subscales, and values of mother and father for family support total and subscales) and 1 between factor (intervention group, with values of experimental and control). Although all possible main and interaction effects were included in each model, only the effects that included the factor for the intervention group were assessed for significance; this assessment was made as a control for overall type I error rate, because this decreased the number of comparisons made. This intervention factor was chosen as the focus of the analysis because the purpose of the study was to evaluate the effect of the therapeutic conversation intervention. In addition, the main effect of intervention was considered for significance only in the case of nonsignificant interaction terms involving this factor; this strategy is necessary because it is not possible to accurately interpret a main effect in the presence of a significant interaction effect. Another strategy to limit type I error was to consider only the post hoc pairwise differences that were preplanned: in particular, the only comparisons made were between 2 levels of a given factor with the other factor(s) fixed. Post hoc analysis was made using Fisher least significant difference procedure for pairwise comparisons. Data analysis was conducted using SAS for Windows, version 9.3; an α level of 0.05 was used throughout.

Ethical Issues

The study was conducted with approval from the Scientific Ethical Board (68/2008) at LUH and with the approval from the Chief Executive of Nursing and Medicine at LUH. This study was also reported to the Data Protection Committee in Iceland (S4118/2008).

RESULTS

There were slightly more boys in the study than girls, particularly in the control group ($P = .05$ for the group comparison; see **Table 1**). Most children were between the ages of 13 and 18 years. Fathers participated from about half of the 31 study families. Most parents were between the ages of 31 and 50 years and were either married or cohabitating. All parents had at least a high school education, with about half also having university education. Most had family income less than 600,000 Icelandic kroners per month. There were no differences between the experimental and control groups on these demographic characteristics except for gender of child.

The illness characteristics and environmental variables are displayed in **Table 2**. Most parents reported their child's asthma as mild or moderate and nearly all had used inhaled steroids during the previous 12 months. More than half had visited the emergency room during the previous 12 months, with a higher percentage in the control group ($P = .04$). Most had received information/education about asthma, although fewer than half responded that they needed support from professionals (about their child's asthma) right now. None of the participating families belonged to an asthma support group at the time of the study. Few participants reported exposure to the potential triggers of secondhand smoke and pets. Only 1 child was exposed to secondhand smoke in the home and 5 children were exposed outside the home; only 1 child had a pet in the home. There were no differences between the 2 intervention groups on prevalence of these potential triggers.

Perceived Family Support

As shown in **Table 3**, there were few differences at baseline (time 1) for either perceived family support or asthma QOL between the experimental and control groups. Although those in the experimental group tended to have more positive assessments at baseline for these measures compared with those in the control group, the group comparisons were only significant among fathers. Fathers in the experimental group rated overall family support and the cognitive support subscale of this measure as higher than did fathers in the control group. In addition, fathers in the experimental group rated the worry subscale of the asthma QOL measure more positively than did fathers in the control group. The comparisons between experimental and control groups for mothers and for children were not significant.

Perceived QOL

For the 3 indicators of family support and 5 indicators of asthma QOL, the main effect on the experimental group either was not significant or was not interpretable, because interactions involving this factor were significant (**Table 4**). For the treatment problems subscale of the asthma QOL measure, there was a significant interaction between experimental group and family member. The post hoc analysis indicated that children

Table 2
Illness characteristics and environmental variables of families of children and adolescents with asthma who received the therapeutic conversation intervention (N = 31 families; n = 31 mothers; n = 15 fathers; n = 31 children)

Illness or Environmental Variable	Experimental Group		Control Group		Test Statistic	
	n	%	n	%	χ^2	P value
Asthma severity						
Mild	7	46.7	4	28.6	3.85	.1
Moderate	8	53.3	7	50.0		
Severe	0	0.0	3	21.4		
Used inhaled steroid within the last 12 mo						
Yes	15	100.0	13	81.3	a	.2
No	0	0.0	3	18.7		
Visit the emergency room within the last 12 mo						
Yes	7	46.7	13	81.3	4.04	.04
No	8	53.3	3	18.7		
Received information now about asthma						
Yes	10	66.7	14	87.5	a	.2
No	5	33.3	2	12.5		
Need support from health care professional						
Yes	4	26.7	6	37.5	a	.7
No	11	73.3	10	62.5		
Belong to an asthma support group						
Yes	0	0.0	0	0.0		
No	15	100.0	16	100.0		
Secondhand smoke exposure inside the home						
Yes	0	0.0	1	6.3	a	>.9
No	15	100.0	15	93.7		
Secondhand smoke exposure outside the home						
Yes	2	13.3	3	18.7	a	>.9
No	13	86.7	13	81.3		
Pets in the home						
Yes	1	6.7	0	0.0	a	.5
No	14	93.3	16	100.0		

[a] Fisher exact test is used when cells have expected counts less than 5; this test calculates a P value but not a test statistic.

in the experimental group had significantly more positive scores for this outcome, compared with mothers in this group, fathers in this group, and children in the control group. In addition, mothers in the control group scored higher (more positively) on this measure, compared with fathers in the control group. None of the interactions between experimental group and time were significant, but the 3-way interaction (experimental group*family member*time) was significant for the summary score and 2 subscales of the family support measure; none of the asthma QOL indicators showed this phenomenon (see **Table 4**).

The post hoc analyses for the significant 3-way interactions are arrayed in **Table 5**. For each of the family support measures, there was a significant increase from time 1 to time 2 for mothers in the experimental group. Whereas mothers in the 2 groups did not differ on these 3 measures at time 1, mothers in the experimental group significantly exceeded mothers in the control group at time 2 for each of the 3. Although there was a significant difference between fathers in the experimental group and

Table 3
Two-sample t tests for mothers, fathers, and children with asthma at time 1 (before intervention)

Variables	Mothers (n = 31)				Fathers (n = 15)				Children (n = 31)			
	EG Mean (SD)	CG Mean (SD)	t	P value	EG Mean (SD)	CG Mean (SD)	t	P value	EG Mean (SD)	CG Mean (SD)	t	P value
Family support	26.2 (17.1)	19.1 (11.9)	1.35	.2	37.6 (16.7)	19.5 (11.1)	2.50	.03				
Cognitive support	11.5 (6.8)	7.8 (5.2)	1.72	.1	16.9 (6.0)	7.9 (4.7)	3.26	.01				
Emotional support	14.7 (10.8)	11.4 (6.9)	1.03	.3	20.7 (12.9)	11.6 (6.7)	1.75	.1				
Asthma QOL	75.4 (12.5)	74.8 (14.9)	0.11	.9	83.0 (5.0)	71.3 (16.4)	1.92	.1	79.3 (11.4)	67.9 (20.8)	1.91	.1
Asthma symptoms	70.6 (17.0)	67.9 (20.3)	0.40	.7	83.1 (9.4)	65.9 (20.1)	2.06	.1	69.7 (13.4)	60.4 (19.8)	1.52	.1
Treatment problems	78.9 (12.4)	82.4 (14.8)	0.70	.5	84.7 (8.3)	76.4 (14.7)	1.32	.2	86.7 (11.6)	76.1 (19.8)	1.82	.1
Worry	83.3 (17.5)	73.4 (23.2)	1.33	.2	90.5 (8.9)	68.8 (20.8)	2.56	.02	89.4 (16.5)	76.6 (28.1)	1.57	.1
Communication	71.7 (23.7)	74.0 (28.7)	0.24	.8	69.0 (36.2)	75.0 (29.2)	0.35	.7	77.2 (25.7)	56.3 (40.3)	1.71	.1

Abbreviations: CG, control group; EG, experimental group; SD, standard deviation.

Sigurdardottir et al

Table 4
F values and significance of intervention of main and interaction effects for repeated measures analysis of variance models[a]

Outcome	Intervention (Main Effect)		Intervention[a] (Family Member)		Intervention[a] (Time)		3-Way Interaction	
	F	P	F	P	F	P	F	P
Family support	6.0	.02	<0.1	.9	0.1	.8	**5.8**[b]	**.03**
Cognitive support	9.2	.005	0.1	.7	<0.1	.9	**5.4**[b]	**.03**
Emotional support	3.7	.06	0.1	.7	<0.1	.9	**5.0**[b]	**.04**
Asthma QOL	2.3	.1	2.6	.8	0.1	.8	0.3	.7
Asthma symptoms	2.3	.1	0.5	.6	<0.1	.8	0.9	.4
Treatment problems	1.3	.3	**5.6**[c]	**.007**	0.2	.7	<0.1	>.9
Worry	3.1	.09	0.4	.7	<0.1	.8	0.3	.8
Communication	1.9	.3	1.2	.3	0.8	.4	0.6	.5

[a] Significant effects bolded.
[b] Means and post hoc comparisons for the significant 3-way interaction for family support and subscales given in **Table 5**.
[c] Post hoc comparisons show that children in the treatment group had higher scores than both mothers in the treatment group (P = .002) and fathers in the treatment group (P = .04); mothers in the control group had higher scores than fathers in the control group (P = .05); children in the treatment group had higher scores than children in the control group (P = .02).

Table 5

Means, standard deviations, and post hoc comparisons for the 3-way interaction (treatment group*parent*time) for the family support scale and subscales (N = 46 parents)

Participant Subgroup	Family Support (Total Score)		Family Support (Cognitive)		Family Support (Emotional)	
	Time 1 Mean (SD)	Time 2 Mean (SD)	Time 1 Mean (SD)	Time 2 Mean (SD)	Time 1 Mean (SD)	Time 2 Mean (SD)
Mothers, experimental group (n = 15)	26.2 (17.1)[a]	35.7 (18.4)[a,b]	11.5 (6.8)[a,c]	15.3 (6.3)[a,b]	14.7 (10.8)[a]	20.4 (12.6)[a,b]
Mothers, control group (n = 16)	19.1 (11.9)	18.9 (7.2)[a,b]	7.8 (5.2)	8.4 (4.5)[b]	11.4 (6.9)	10.4 (3.1)[b]
Fathers, experimental group (n = 7)	37.6 (16.7)[d]	32.2 (18.3)	16.9 (6.0)[c,d]	14.7 (5.5)	20.7 (12.9)	17.5 (13.5)
Fathers, control group (n = 8)	19.5 (11.1)[d]	25.8 (11.5)	7.9 (4.7)[d]	10.6 (4.3)	11.6 (6.7)	15.2 (7.3)

[a] Significant increase among experimental mothers from time 1 to time 2: $P = .002$ for total, $P = .002$ for cognitive, $P = .01$ for emotional.
[b] Significant difference between experimental and control mothers at time 2: $P = .002$ for total, $P = .002$ for cognitive, $P = .004$ for emotional.
[c] Significant difference between experimental mothers and fathers at time 1: $P = .01$ for cognitive.
[d] Significant difference between experimental and control fathers at time 1: $P = .04$ for total, $P = .007$ for cognitive.

fathers in the control group at time 1 for both total family support and the cognitive subscale, this difference was not found at the time 2 survey. Experimental mothers scored significantly lower than experimental fathers at time 1, but only for the measure of cognitive support.

DISCUSSION

The main findings from this study, as determined from the repeated measures analysis of variance models, indicate that the added benefit of the brief FAM-TC intervention for families of children and adolescents with asthma is promising. Mothers in the experimental group reported significantly higher family support both for the total scale as well as for the subscales of cognitive and emotional support over time. In addition, the mothers in the experimental group also reported significantly higher perception on family support and significantly higher scores on the cognitive and emotional subscales of the family support scale after the intervention compared with the mothers who received treatment as usual. This finding about the benefit of the brief FAM-TC intervention for the mothers (typically the primary caregivers of the children in this study) is helpful for clinicians and supports the need for such a family-level psychosocial and educational intervention in clinical settings. Even although the mothers in this study, who primarily were either married or cohabiting with their partner, typically had a child with moderate or mild asthma and had been dealing with the asthma condition for a reasonably long period of time (on average for 8 years), these mothers found the components of the 2-session FAM-TC intervention, such as offering caregiver support, offering easy-to-read literature and offering information and professional opinion about the asthma situation, to be of added benefit for them and their families.

Among the children who participated, mainly preadolescents or adolescents, for the subscale of problems with asthma treatment on the asthma QOL scale, there was a significant decline between preintervention and postintervention for children whose parents were in the experimental group, relative to the children who had parents in the control group. Further, the children of parents who received the intervention also reported significantly fewer problems with asthma treatment than did their mothers and their fathers. This finding on the benefit of the 2-session FAM-TC intervention for the children of parents in the intervention group is new and exciting. The finding that the children of the parents in the experimental group perceived they had fewer problems with their asthma treatment after their parents had received the FAM-TC intervention agrees with the emphasis in the Calgary Models.[9] According to Wright and Leahey,[9] when therapeutic conversation interventions are developed to meet the needs of the families, and when there is a fit between the clinical nurse specialist (the clinicians who offer the intervention) and the parents, then children with chronic asthma can benefit from the interventions. Further, these findings are in harmony with findings reported by Burkhart and colleagues,[17] who found asthma was better controlled when school-aged children and their families followed recommended asthma treatment, and that this in turn improved children's QOL. In addition, the findings that children reported significantly fewer problems with asthma treatment compared with their parents' perception are in agreement with findings reported by Rayens and colleagues,[22] who found that American parents of teenagers with asthma tended to underrate their children's QOL compared with the adolescents' evaluations of their own asthma QOL.

The fathers in the intervention group did not differ significantly from fathers in the usual care group at postintervention on perceived family support, including the total scale and the subscales of cognitive or emotional support. However, before the intervention, the fathers in the experimental group reported significantly higher family support and significantly higher cognitive support (the subscale of the family support scale) than the fathers in the control group. The findings on the lack of benefit of the 2-session FAM-TC intervention, for fathers in the experimental group, are contradictory to the theoretic framework that guided the study. Wright and Leahey[9] have emphasized that both parents in the family can benefit from such a therapeutic conversation intervention. One explanation for the lack of significant findings for the fathers is that the fathers in the experimental group scored significantly higher before intervention on the family support scale and on the cognitive support subscale than the fathers in the control group, which may suggest that these fathers already perceived family support positively. In addition, the sample of fathers was small and all of them worked full-time outside the home, which could have resulted in increased difficulty both in recruiting fathers to participate in the study (as shown by lower numbers of father participants) and perhaps in establishing rapport with the fathers who did participate, given that many were likely to be secondary caregivers. In addition, the 2-session FAM-TC intervention might not have met the needs of the fathers, because they may need to have either a more in-depth intervention or a totally different one, focusing on different components.

The preintervention result regarding the gender differences between the mothers and the fathers in the experimental group, with higher scores on the total score and cognitive subscale of the family support subscale among fathers compared with mothers, is noteworthy. This finding may be explained because most of the mothers were primary caregivers of the preadolescents and adolescents with asthma, which might have resulted in a greater need for specific information regarding asthma management of teenagers, even before the parents participated in the intervention. On the other hand, fathers, who typically were the secondary caregiver, may have been more satisfied with their asthma management knowledge before the intervention. In addition, even although most of the parents in both groups indicated that their child had used inhaled steroids within the last year, most of the parents in the control group and half of the parents in the experimental group reported that they had visited the emergency room within the same interval of time. Many of these parents did not make this indication before the intervention, and they were now in need of support from health care professionals even although none of these families belonged to an asthma support group. Advanced nurses caring for families of children and teenagers with asthma need to be able to assess and to intervene on a family system level, because this provides the parents with the support that they need in their daily caregiving activities.

LIMITATION

The primary limitation of this exploratory study is the sample size. Although 77 individuals participated, they represent the members of 31 families, with 15 families in the experimental group and 16 in the control group. An additional limitation is that the families were not randomly assigned to experimental group, given the limited availability of the interventionist. The steps taken to minimize the impact of these limitations were to limit the number of comparisons made (in an effort to minimize the overall type I error) and to verify that the experimental and control groups were comparable at baseline, with few differences found among the demographic or outcome variables. Future studies in this area will benefit from having a larger sample size and families randomly assigned to the experimental or control group.

SUMMARY

The findings regarding the benefits of the 2-session theory-based FAM-TC intervention underscore the importance of such interventions when offering evidence-based practice to families of children and adolescents with asthma. Knowing that the components of this short-term educational and psychosocial intervention benefited the mothers in the experimental group, when compared with the mothers in the control group, is of special interest to clinicians who are often working on a busy pediatric unit, with limited time for each family. Further, knowing that the children with asthma who had parents in the experimental group reported fewer problems with their asthma treatment in the previous month when compared with the children who had parents in the control group adds to the validation of the short-term FAM-TC intervention for these families. This finding provides further support for offering evidence-based health care services; the implication is that administrators and advanced nurse practitioners need to implement meaningful research into clinical practices by systematically supporting knowledge translation into clinical settings. Further research focusing on the benefits of the intervention and on the relationships with family functioning as well as with satisfaction with the health care services is needed. Furthermore, research on how the intervention can be maintained in a regular clinical practice is important; as well as studying the specific needs for families of such an intervention based on the time from diagnoses of asthma and on the age range of the children with asthma.

ACKNOWLEDGMENTS

The authors would like to express their sincere thanks to the children, adolescents, and parents who participated in this study for sharing their experiences. We would also like to give special thanks to Mariu Gudnadottir RN, MSc and Tonie Sörensen RN, BSc, nurses at the Children's Hospital at LUH in Iceland, for their important and valuable contribution of the study. They participated in the data collection and conducted the therapeutic conversations with the families.

REFERENCES

1. Akinbami LJ, Moorman JE, Garbe PL, et al. Status of childhood asthma in the United States, 1980–2007. Pediatrics 2009;123(Suppl 3):S131–45.
2. Global Initiative for Asthma. Global strategy for asthma management and prevention. 2011. Available at: http://www.ginasthma.org/. Accessed August 20, 2012.
3. Clausen M, Kristjansson S, Haraldsson A, et al. High prevalence of allergic diseases and sensitization in a low allergen country. Acta Paediatr 2008;97(9):1216–20.
4. Flores G, Abreu M, Tomany-Korman S, et al. Keeping children with asthma out of hospitals: parents' and physicians' perspectives on how pediatric asthma hospitalizations can be prevented. Pediatrics 2005;116(4):957–65.
5. Coffman JM, Cabana MD, Halpin HA, et al. Effects of asthma education on children's use of acute care services: a meta-analysis. Pediatrics 2008;121(3):575–86.
6. Boyd M, Lasserson TJ, McKean MC, et al. Interventions for educating children who are at risk of asthma-related emergency department attendance. Cochrane Database Syst Rev 2009;(4).
7. Mansour ME, Lanphear BP, DeWitt TG. Barriers to asthma care in urban children: parent perspectives. Pediatrics 2000;106(3):512–9.

8. Leahey M, Svavarsdottir EK. Implementing family nursing: how do we translate knowledge into clinical practice? J Fam Nurs 2009;15(4):445–60.

9. Wright LM, Leahey M. Nurses and families: a guide to family assessment and intervention, vol. 5. Philadelphia: FA Davis; 2009.

10. Wright LM, Bell JM. Beliefs and illness: a model for healing. Calgary (Alberta, Canada): 4th Floor Press; 2009.

11. Svavarsdottir EK, Sigurdardottir AO. Implementing family nursing in general pediatric nursing practice. The circularity between knowledge translation and clinical practice. In: Svavarsdottir EK, Jonsdottir H, editors. Family nursing in action. Reykjavik (Iceland): University of Iceland Press; 2011. p. 161–84.

12. Åstedt-Kurki P, Kaunonen M. Family nursing interventions in Finland: benefits for families. In: Svavarsdottir EK, Jonsdottir H, editors. Family nursing in action. Reykjavik (Iceland): University of Iceland Press; 2011. p. 115–59.

13. Svavarsdottir EK, Tryggvadottir GB, Sigurdardottir AO. Knowledge translation in family nursing: does a short-term therapeutic conversation intervention benefit families of children and adolescents in a hospital setting? Findings from the Landspitali University Hospital family nursing implementation. J Fam Nurs 2012;18(3):303–27.

14. Bell JM, Wright LM. The illness beliefs model: creating practice knowledge in family system nursing for families experiencing illness. In: Svavarsdottir EK, Jonsdottir H, editors. Family nursing in action. . Reykjavik (Iceland): University of Iceland Press; 2011. p. 15–51.

15. Long KA, Ewing LJ, Cohen S, et al. Preliminary evidence for the feasibility of a stress management intervention for 7- to 12-year-olds with asthma. J Asthma 2011;48(2):162–70.

16. Bloomberg GR, Banister C, Sterkel R, et al. Socioeconomic, family, and pediatric practice factors that affect level of asthma control. Pediatrics 2009;123(3):829–35.

17. Burkhart PV, Rayens MK, Oakley MG. Effect of peak flow monitoring on child asthma quality of life. J Pediatr Nurs 2012;27(1):18–25.

18. Svavarsdottir EK, Garwick AW, Anderson LS, et al. The international school nurse asthma project: barriers related to asthma management in schools. J Adv Nurs 2012. [Epub ahead of print]. http://dx.doi.org/10.1111/j.1365-2648.2012.06107.x.

19. Juniper EF, Guyatt GH, Feeny DH, et al. Measuring quality of life in children with asthma. Qual Life Res 1996;5(1):35–46.

20. Varni JW, Limbers CA. The pediatric quality of life inventory: measuring pediatric health-related quality of life from the perspective of children and their parents. Pediatr Clin North Am 2009;56(4):843–63.

21. Everhart RS, Fiese BH. Asthma severity and child quality of life in pediatric asthma: a systematic review. Patient Educ Couns 2009;75(2):162–8.

22. Rayens MK, Svavarsdottir EK, Burkart PV. Cultural differences in parent-adolescent agreement on the adolescent's asthma-related quality of life. Pediatr Nurs 2011;37(6):311–9.

23. Konradsdottir E, Svavarsdottir EK. How effective is a short-term educational and support intervention for families of an adolescent with type 1 diabetes? J Spec Pediatr Nurs 2011;16(4):295–304.

24. Svavarsdottir EK, Sigurdardottir A. The feasibility of offering a family level intervention to parents of children with cancer. Scand J Caring Sci 2005;19(4):368–72.

25. Svavarsdottir EK, Sigurdardottir AO. Developing a family-level intervention for families of children with cancer. Oncol Nurs Forum 2006;33(5):983–90.

26. Holtslander L. Clinical application of the 15-minute family interview: addressing the needs of postpartum families. J Fam Nurs 2005;11(1):5–18.

27. Legrow K, Rossen BE. Development of professional practice based on a family systems nursing framework: nurses' and families' experiences. J Fam Nurs 2005; 11(1):38–58.
28. Martinez AM, D'Artois D, Rennick JE. Does the 15-minute (or less) family interview influence family nursing practice? J Fam Nurs 2007;13(2):157–78.
29. Kamban SW, Svavarsdottir EK. Does a therapeutic conversation intervention in an acute paediatric setting make a difference for families of children with bronchiolitis caused by respiratory syncytial virus RSV? J Clin Nurs, in press.
30. Varni JW, Burwinkle TM, Rapoff MA, et al. The PedsQL™ in pediatric asthma: reliability and validity of the Pediatric Quality of Life Inventory™ generic core scales and asthma module. J Behav Med 2004;27(3):297–318.
31. Sveinbjarnardottir EK, Svavarsdottir EK, Hrafnkelsson B. Psychometric development of the Iceland-family perceived support questionnaire (ICE-FPSQ). J Fam Nurs 2012;18(3):328–52.

Health Care Autonomy in Children with Chronic Conditions
Implications for Self-Care and Family Management

Barbara L. Beacham, MSN, RN[a],*, Janet A. Deatrick, PhD, FAAN[b]

KEYWORDS

- Child • Development • Chronic health conditions • Family management • Self-care
- Autonomy

KEY POINTS

- Autonomy in health care situations usually is one of the last contexts in which autonomy is expressed, typically in late adolescence.
- Self-care for children with chronic conditions incorporates self-care maintenance, self-care monitoring, and self-care management.
- Current care guidelines stipulate that health care providers and family caregivers need to ensure that children with chronic conditions master developmentally appropriate knowledge and skills regarding their disease.
- School-aged children between the ages of 8 and 13 years with chronic conditions are becoming more knowledgeable about their disease and acquiring more skills to support their management activities.
- The development of health care autonomy requires appropriate family management because self-care develops from parent-focused care, to joint/cooperative/shared care, to child-determined care.
- Supporting the development of health care autonomy in school-aged children with chronic health conditions also supports the development of self-care and more optimal outcomes throughout adolescence.
- During adolescence, children with chronic health conditions may experience a decline in management outcomes.

This work was supported by grant nos. F31NR11524 and T32NR007100 from the National Institutes of Health, National Institute of Nursing Research and by a grant from the Sigma Theta Tau Xi Chapter, University of Pennsylvania.
The authors have nothing to disclose.
[a] Center for Health Equity Research, University of Pennsylvania School of Nursing, Room 243 (2Lower) Claire M. Fagin Hall, 418 Curie Boulevard, Philadelphia, PA 19104-4217, USA;
[b] Center for Health Equity Research, University of Pennsylvania School of Nursing, Room 223 (2Lower) Claire M. Fagin Hall, 418 Curie Boulevard, Philadelphia, PA 19104-4217, USA
* Corresponding author.
E-mail address: blynne@nursing.upenn.edu

http://dx.doi.org/10.1016/j.cnur.2013.01.010
0029-6465/13/$ – see front matter © 2013 Elsevier Inc. All rights reserved.
nursing.theclinics.com

More than half of all Americans have at least 1 chronic health condition,[1] and 1 in 5 households have a child who has a chronic health condition.[2] Because most of these children now survive into adulthood,[3] their transition to self-care and eventually to adult health care is on the clinical, research, and policy agendas for many professional, advocacy, and governmental groups.[4–6] Although common sense links child development, family issues, and the acquisition of self-care, a gap exists regarding how the components can be integrated into a model to guide nursing practice.

Health care autonomy is a developmental key that links family management and self-care. Autonomy is the ability to evaluate options, make a decision and define a goal, feel confident about those decisions, and develop strategies to meet the goal.[7] Health care autonomy refers to the ability to evaluate options, make decisions and define health-related goals, have the confidence to stand by those decisions, and develop strategies to meet those health-related goals. Autonomy in health care situations for children is usually one of the last contexts in which autonomy is expressed, typically in late adolescence.[8,9]

The general importance of autonomy is highlighted along with other factors, including family management and skills for self-management, in a social-ecological model of readiness to transition (SMART) to adult health care for children with chronic conditions proposed by Schwartz and colleagues.[10] They explicitly indicate the importance of autonomy (developmental maturity), family management styles, and self-management to the transition process. The developmentally appropriate level of autonomy for the child is mentioned as a facilitator of the transition process. For all concerned (including the child and the family), family management goals that facilitate the child's autonomy and successful transition to adult care are necessary. More specifically, the family members and the family as a unit need to believe that the child is capable (ie, child identity) and that the child will be able to care for himself/herself in the future (ie, future expectations).[11] In addition, Schwartz and colleagues[10] point out that children who successfully transition must have disease self-management skills and parents need to be effective at supporting such skills.

The purposes of this article are (1) to describe a developmental and family-based model of health care autonomy that incorporates self-care and family management and (2) to apply the model to 2 case studies to highlight how it can be applied to nursing practice and the possibility of nursing research.

DEVELOPMENT OF HEALTH CARE AUTONOMY

The development of autonomy is integral to the development of self-care in children with chronic health conditions. As the model in **Fig. 1** depicts, health care autonomy, family management, and self-care provide the foundation for child health and well-being. Examining these concepts can provide a basis for understanding the challenges of incorporating the management of a chronic condition into transitioning to young adulthood and how nursing care can best support this process.

The left-hand side of the model depicts the key components required for development of autonomy. Autonomy readiness is assessed both by the parent and by the child, separately and based on the feedback they get from one another. It is these individual assessments, along with the interactions between the child and parent, that provide the foundation for family management of the chronic health condition and the development of self-care within the child. The optimal outcomes of the process are health and well-being of the child and increasing health care autonomy.

Chronic health conditions can lead to decreased well-being for the child in terms of missed school days and opportunities for social interactions and activities, as well as

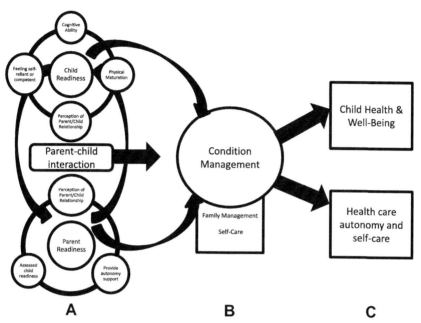

Fig. 1. Development of health care autonomy (*A*) Parent-child Autonomy Readiness Factors include those areas the child and parent assess independently and in interaction with one another to determine readiness to increase child health care autonomy for condition management. (*B*) Interaction/Activity considers the condition management, both from the family and child. (*C*) Child outcome examines the child health and well-being as well as the child autonomy and self-care.

lost productivity, poor health, lost wages, and increased medical expenses for parents.[12,13] Families of children with chronic health conditions face the challenge of managing all facets of the condition early in the child's life and then transitioning the management responsibility to the child. Therefore, by understanding the process of developing health care autonomy, and the key components for both the child and the parent, health care providers can help to maximize child health outcomes.

HEALTH CARE AUTONOMY

Autonomy is a complex developmental construct; it is instrumental in the transition from childhood to adulthood. Successful autonomy can be assessed by examining decision making, relationships, influence on others, and perception of competence, control, and responsibility.[7] It is often believed to be synonymous with independence and self-reliance.

In a study of decision-making autonomy, Smetana and colleagues[8] identified 4 different domains of autonomy: prudential, conventional, multifaceted, and personal. Each domain reflects a different context for autonomy development, with prudential (decisions regarding health and safety, e.g., when/if to smoke cigarettes, drink alcohol) and personal (decisions regarding the state of one's body, privacy) being especially relevant to the child with a chronic health condition. Each domain deals with different issues and therefore autonomy develops in each domain over time but at different times and rates. The study also found that mothers and children had different perceptions about when the child should or did have increased autonomy in each area.

Children with chronic health conditions need to develop autonomy within these domains specifically related to the management of their chronic health condition. As stated earlier, autonomy over health-related issues (prudential) typically occurs late in adolescence,[8,9] but we often expect children with chronic health conditions to master these tasks earlier. Helping children master all the components of self-care requires a well-constructed plan over many years and requires the support and buy in of the child and family.[5]

FAMILY MANAGEMENT FOR CHILDREN WITH CHRONIC CONDITIONS

Family management, how families actively organize, integrate, and accomplish tasks related to the chronic health condition in the child,[11] supports the health and well-being of the child. The 3 components and 8 dimensions of family management identified by Knafl and colleagues[11] highlight the areas and issues that families and practitioners need to consider. In the first component, definition of the situation, there are 4 dimensions. The family view of the child with a chronic health condition (child identity) and the view of the condition itself (view of condition) are the first 2 dimensions and are the foundation of family management. The next two dimensions develop from this understanding as the parents also assess the ease or difficulty they have in carrying out the recommended treatments (management mindset) and the extent to which they have shared views of the child, condition and approach to condition management (parental mutuality). The second conceptual component, management behaviors, identifies 2 dimensions, the parenting philosophy regarding condition management (parenting philosophy) and the ability of the parents and child to have a routine and strategies for condition management (management approach).[11] The third component, perceived consequences, is comprised of 2 dimensions, the parents' assessment and satisfaction with how condition management has been incorporated into family life (family focus) and the parents assessment of the future for both the child and the family (future expectation).

Family management changes over the course of a child's life as the child develops the skills, cognitive ability, and social confidence to manage their own health care activities. The authors of the model, developed primarily from the parents' perspective, have encouraged researchers to expand its use to other populations. A study of adolescents with spina bifida demonstrated the value of adolescents' perceptions of how they manage their condition with their family.[14] The adolescents' description of condition management performed by themselves or their families was consistent with the dimensions and components within the family management model. In addition, self-management as well as the shared responsibility of care between the adolescent and the parent, was highlighted.

Moving the science forward requires research regarding the children's perceptions about how their families manage within the context of their own self-care, because the child is both a recipient of family management and a participant with the family as they manage. Only then can the interplay of the family and child be examined, recognizing that some of the components or dimensions of family management may remain stagnant and may not support the development of the child. Optimal family management would transition most of the condition management to the child as they grow and develop, while maintaining health outcomes.

SELF-CARE FOR CHILDREN WITH CHRONIC CONDITIONS

Riegel and colleagues'[15(p195)] middle-range theory of self-care was created from experience with adults who have heart failure. The theory defines self-care as "a process of maintaining health through health promoting practices and managing illness." The 3 components of the theory, self-care maintenance, self-care monitoring, and self-care management, delineate self-care and identify areas to consider when teaching children and their families.

Self-care maintenance is the behaviors used by patients with chronic conditions to maintain physical and emotional stability.[15] For children, the family, and health care provider, determining when the child is developmentally able to perform these behaviors is important when considering transitioning from an emphasis on parental agency in family management to child agency and self-care.

Self-care monitoring, the second component, is the process of observation or self-reflection to identify changes in signs and symptoms.[15] Again, the ability to attend to this process depends on the child's developmental ability and self-awareness. This component is most overlooked when considering a child's ability to perform self-care and may be a reason for a decline in outcomes during adolescence.

The third component of the model, self-care management, is defined as a response to the signs and symptoms when they occur.[15] Taking appropriate action requires knowledge of the options available, availability of the treatments required, and the physical ability and the psychosocial maturity to act. The child may have the knowledge, but not the maturity to act when faced with having to show weakness in front of friends or classmates. Both components of management are crucial when preparing the child for self-care activities.

This conceptualization of self-care provides a novel way to examine all the components of self-care that may be applicable for children with chronic health conditions and their families as they navigate the process of maintaining the health of the child. **Table 1** demonstrates the way the original framework may be adapted to include children and families. This adapted model is used as a template to examine the care components that families provide and transition to children over time.

Self-care for children with chronic health conditions is a joint effort between the family/parents and the child. Learning self-care practices begins as a parent/caregiver driven effort when the child is young, with the goal of transitioning to a child driven effort as the child becomes a young adult. The process of transitioning can be seen in everyday self-care activities, such as oral care. When a child is born and throughout infancy, the parent/caregiver is responsible for maintaining oral care. As the child develops the ability to handle a toothbrush, they are given a toothbrush; which they basically chew on. The parent perseveres and handles the actual tooth brushing while the child is learning about brushing his/her own teeth. The child observes and experiences the parents' tooth brushing and alters their own actions with each attempt. Once the child is able to brush his/her own teeth, the parent still follows up to ensure they are doing a good job. Over time the child proves that they are able to brush his/her own teeth. Tooth brushing become a child driven self-care activity, although the parent may still handle making appointments and acute situations. Physical ability is 1 component that drives the transfer of care from the parent to child; another is the child's ability to act autonomously.

The level of self-care a child is capable of depends on several factors. Knowledge of the disease and treatment regime, which is part of self-care maintenance, along with the age of the child have been attributed to skill mastery.[16] But skill mastery is only 1 part of self-care. A study of children with asthma found that symptom recognition, the ability to identify changes early, and intervene appropriately are described by older children but not younger ones.[17] This study also found that older children with asthma were more adept at self-care management and were able to manage an asthma attack independently, whereas younger children required assistance and all children lacked

Table 1
Adaption of a self-care model

Self-care	Definition[a]	Adaptation for Child/Family	Examples of Self-care in Action
Self-care	Process of maintaining health through health-promoting practices and managing illness	Family management to maintain health-promoting practices and managing illness; believes that the child will be or is capable and expects the child to care for self in the future	Transition from parental agency and family management to child agency and self-care
Self-care maintenance	Behaviors performed to improve well-being, preserve health, or to maintain physical and emotional stability	Behaviors performed by the child and/or family to improve well-being, preserve health, or to maintain physical and emotional stability	Daily flossing and brushing teeth. Reduced sugar intake. Biannual checkups
Self-care monitoring	Process of routine, vigilant body monitoring, surveillance, or body listening	Process of routine, vigilant body monitoring, surveillance, or body listening by the child and family	Awareness of tooth and gum status, sensitivity to hot/cold, bleeding, pain, need to brush teeth after eating and food sticks to or between your teeth
Self-care management	Involves evaluation of changes in physical and emotional signs and symptoms to determine if action is needed	The evaluation of changes in physical and emotional signs and symptoms by the child and/or family to determine if action is needed	Evaluation of tooth/gum pain and deciding to call the dentist, brush, or floss as needed in addition to twice a day

[a] Definitions from Riegel and colleagues.[15(pp 195–6)]

the knowledge required to avoid asthma triggers and prevent an attack.[17] This finding is not surprising because symptom recognition is inherent in self-care monitoring and is a more sophisticated skill.

As children get older, studies have found that there is a decrease in self-care (medical adherence) for children with chronic conditions during adolescence resulting in a decrease in well-being.[18] For example, a 4-year longitudinal study of children with diabetes found that age was related to a decline in metabolic control.[19] In addition, self-care behaviors (maintenance) also declined over this period. Peer relationships were a risk factor for poor control. The investigators posited that some of the deterioration may have been related to decreased parental monitoring, supervision, and overall involvement in the diabetes management. In addition, parents may have decreased monitoring and direct involvement based on the observation that their school-aged children seemed to be autonomous because they were adherent with self-care maintenance. Attempting to reestablish monitoring and parental agency or control with an adolescent often fails. What may not have been so obvious when the parent decreased monitoring is that the adolescent did not have the requisite skills regarding health care autonomy that are involved in self-care monitoring and management. This exemplifies the dilemma faced by families during the transition of responsibilities. Without adequate training, development, and oversight, the child is not being prepared for success in all areas necessary for successful condition management. If parents totally abdicate and withdraw support and monitoring, trying to regain parental control may not be successful and outcomes may suffer. Therefore, the school-age period is an extremely important but delicate time of preparation and transition.

SELF-CARE, FAMILY MANAGEMENT, AND HEALTH CARE AUTONOMY

Thus, the ability to practice self-care is dependent on the child's developmental stage. Just as the child needed the dexterity to hold a tooth brush and understanding not to swallow the toothpaste, children need the cognitive, physical, and psychosocial abilities to be autonomous with condition management. When children are too young (not developmentally able) to successfully handle all the demands of self-care, the family shoulders the condition management responsibilities. The family must optimally include the child as an active participant and allow them to observe the process used to make decisions. By actively participating in a developmentally appropriate manner, the child learns the thought processes, and can begin to understand the decision-making processes that are behind the skills and medical regimes they may already be doing.

For autonomy to develop, both the child and the parent need to be prepared. For the child, readiness to assume more autonomy for health-related matters is dependent on cognitive ability, physical maturation, feelings of competence or self-reliance, and the perception of the parent/child relationship.[20] Somewhat independently, the parent is assessing the child's readiness to assume more autonomy, their own willingness to support autonomy development and relinquish management responsibility, and their perception of the relationship with the child (see **Fig. 1**).

The parent-child interaction determines the management activities and how those activities and decisions can be handled. Not surprisingly, the relationship between the child and parent, along with the family are important components in both the development of autonomy and self-care. Parental supports for the development of autonomy are those behaviors that provide autonomy support, that is, praise and encouragement,[21] as opposed to behaviors aimed at controlling the child or adolescent.[22,23] Maternal separation anxiety decreases as the child grows older, and this allows cognitive autonomy to increase.[24]

Although the child and parent relationship may be harmonious, the perception of autonomy is not always congruent between parents and their children. Butner and colleagues[25] found that adolescents rated their functional autonomy higher than their parents. Although parents had less confidence in the adolescents' ability to act autonomously, they were willing to allow increased autonomy, even though outcomes declined.

Age also plays a role in the development of autonomy. In a study of children with diabetes, age at diagnosis was positively associated with child-only responsibility and negatively associated with parent-only responsibility.[16] Similar findings were made in a study on asthma in which older children showed more autonomous behaviors than younger ones, and parents were the primary decision makers for the younger child.[17] Setting may also be important for school-aged children, because regardless of age, most of them informed an adult when they experienced an asthma attack in a social setting.

Years of experience with a medication or treatment may also influence autonomy. When children had used a pump to deliver their insulin, the more responsible they were regarding knowledge of diabetes management and the less the parents were responsible for pump operations.[16] This study also reported a relationship between age at diagnosis and increased likelihood of the child having independent responsibility for continuous subcutaneous insulin infusion care.

Children mentioned behaviors that were autonomous including taking medications or telling someone when they were sick or having an asthma attack.[17] Taking medication is a multistep task and understanding what it means to the child is important to understanding the degree of autonomy they have. A child may say they take their medication on their own, but the parent provides the medication or reminds them to take it. It is the parent who most likely is still scheduling the doctor appointments and ordering the medication so that it is available for the child to take. The larger task of obtaining the medication and ensuring it is available when and where the child needs it, is typically left up to the parent far beyond the school-age years.

Looking closer at what is known about the development of autonomy and its relation to self-care, it can be seen that there are a couple of assumptions that need to be stated. For children, condition management involves interplay between health care autonomy, family management, and self-care. This relationship depends on the child's development (physical, cognitive, psychological, and social) as well as the parents' and child's assessment of readiness for assuming more responsibility and independence regarding condition management. If the child is to assume more responsibility, the parent must be ready to relinquish some of the control to the child. Relinquishing control, however, does not mean that the parents withdraw entirely from the process. The child needs to be supported in their attempts at autonomously assuming responsibility for self-care, coached through the trials of nonoptimal condition management, encouraged to make good decisions, and appropriately monitored by their parents.[26,27] Family management optimally recognizes that the child needs to develop self-care in all 3 areas, maintenance, monitoring and management. Exploring the development of self-care in the light of emerging autonomy and family management, there are areas for which guidance, oversight, and monitoring may need to continue, even as the child assumes more and more responsibility and autonomy. That is, developing self-care does not mean that there is no longer assistance, advice, and support from the family or others. Successful self-care is not a solitary endeavor and needs to be supported.

Table 2 represents the intersection of health care autonomy, self-care, and family management. Identifying the important factors for autonomy development that can influence the development of self-care can help health care providers to guide parents and children to ease the transitions and minimize changes in outcomes. Understanding how and where family management guides this process for the child identifies areas where support and interventions may be required. The case studies and discussion that follow were developed systematically from **Table 2**. They are intended to highlight some of the areas where families may need guidance and children may need support in light of the knowledge that health care providers have regarding autonomy, self-care, and family management.

CASE STUDY 1

Michael, a 12-year-old boy, lives in a large 4-bedroom house with his mother, father, younger brother, and pet dog. The father works outside the home and the mother maintains the home and coordinates all family activities. She believes the family has enough money to live comfortably and that the health insurance through her husband's job covers most of the medical expenses for the family. Michael does

Table 2
Intersection of autonomy, self-care, and family management

Autonomy Requirements	Self-care Maintenance[a]	Self-care Monitoring[a]	Self-care Management[a]	Family Management[b] Component
Developmental stage	Consider all developmental areas, especially cognitive and psychosocial, Maslow's hierarchy of needs			Child identity Parenting philosophy Family focus
Self-reliance	Is the child confident he/she can do the tasks at hand?	Is the child able to identify the signs and symptoms of condition change and communicate as needed?	Is the child able to decide on the intervention required and take the necessary steps?	Child identity View of the condition Parenting philosophy Management mindset Management approach Future expectation
Physical ability	Does the child have the strength, dexterity, physical attributes necessary to perform the task?	Is the child self-aware of his/her own body to recognize the signs and symptoms of condition change?	Does the child have the strength, dexterity, physical attributes necessary to perform the task?	Child identity
Cognitive ability	Does the child have the cognitive ability required to perform the tasks?	Does the child have the cognitive ability to recognize change in the signs and symptoms?	Can the child make decisions regarding condition management?	Management mindset
Psychosocial ability	Does the child have the support systems in place and the emotional maturity to maintain self-care?			Child identity View of condition Parental mutuality Parenting philosophy
Perception of parent/child relationship	Does the child feel supported and trusted by the parent while they transition and assume more maintenance responsibility?	Is the child listened to when they perceive a change in condition that requires intervention of some sort and are they supported in decision making?	Is the child supported during management attempts and allowed to reflect on different possible courses?	Child identity View of condition Management approach Family focus Future expectations

[a] Adapted from the Self-Care model, Riegel and colleagues.[15]
[b] Adapted from the Family Management Styles Framework, Knafl and colleagues.[11]

well in school; his favorite subjects are mathematics and science. He has friends that he spends time with after school and at weekends. He is involved in sports, plays baseball and basketball, and participates in scouts. He was diagnosed with diabetes when he was 6 years old and thinks that it is no big deal. Sometimes he gets frustrated when he has to stop doing something and check his blood sugar level, but mostly it is okay because "Mom takes care of everything." She handles the daily dispensing of medications, draws up the insulin, and gives Michael his injections. Michael says he tried to draw up his own insulin and give himself the injection when he was 9 years old, but Mom said he did not do it right so she has done it ever since. He thinks that when he is 15 years he might be old enough to draw up the insulin and give himself the injections. He does prick his finger and use the glucometer, but reports the results to Mom, who takes over from there. A chart on the refrigerator shows how much insulin is required for the glucose levels, but Michael is not interested in checking it out, "Mom and Dad tell me what to do and I just do it. It's easier that way."

CASE STUDY 2

Sam is a 12-year-old girl with cystic fibrosis, asthma, and lactose intolerance. She does well in school, likes to play with friends; takes dance lessons, and plays the piano. She and her mother, father, older brother, and sister live in a modest 3-bedroom row home in the city. She shares a bedroom with her sister and has her half of the room decorated in pink and has pictures of current pop musicians on the walls. Sam is able to identify the medications that she takes and knows why she takes them. She is responsible for filling her weekly pill box on Sunday night and then her Mom or Dad checks it for accuracy. She has a small purse that she carries with her when she goes to a friend's home and brings along her enzymes and inhaler. She easily identifies when she needs to take extra enzymes when having a snack and when she has used her emergency inhaler. She usually does not ask or tell anyone about the enzymes, but if she needs to use her inhaler, she usually informs her Mom or other adult because "sometimes it doesn't work and I need something else." She explains how she had chest physiotherapy when she was younger, which she liked and misses because it felt good, but now uses a vest twice a day. She was involved in discussions with the doctor and her Mom regarding sleepovers and said she now uses the acapella (Smiths Medical, St. Paul, MN), "it's easier to take with me and do at a sleepover." She gets frustrated at school when the people in the cafeteria will not let her have a certain food because they think she cannot have it. She tells her Mom when she gets home and the mother calls the school. It works for about a week and then they go back to the old way. She does not see a time when it will be different at school. She is learning to hook herself up to her nightly feeding tube and at first thought it was fun, learning something new. But now it is kind of boring and she prefers when her parents do it as it interrupts her playing before bed.

Although both Michael and Sam are 12 years old, their families treat them differently. Both children know about their condition, but Sam is a much more active participant in her daily care. She has assumed some responsibility in preparing her daily medications but Mom or Dad monitor the activity. She is fairly independent in taking her enzymes before meals and snacks and has autonomy over the activity when visiting with friends. She is being supported to learn new self-care skills, such as attaching herself to the feeding pump for overnight feeds, with the support and direction of her parents. Michael, on the other hand, has not progressed much from his initial task of checking his blood sugar. He is not responsible for recording the results or figuring out how much insulin he requires. He lacked support when he attempted to draw up his own insulin and self-inject, feeling that he was not old enough to do it, and estimates he will be having Mom draw up and inject for another 3 years.

Although Sam is involved in decisions regarding treatment options, Michael has not been involved and cannot explain his recent change in insulin. He has to be reminded to check his blood sugar level before eating a snack at home, and required additional reminding to tell Mom what his blood sugar level was so that she could get the insulin prepared.

Both parents admit to worrying about the children, but Sam's mother says that Sam is going to grow up and have to take care of herself, and although they will always be there for her, she will have to take care of herself someday. They are working toward that day in slow easy steps. Michael's Mom also sees that Michael will need to take care of himself someday, but says that he will have to do it when he is older; "while I'm here and I can do it for him, it allows him to be more like a regular kid. I take care of his diabetes so he doesn't have to think about it."

Although there are no absolutes, Michael's parents are not providing him with the skills and understanding he needs as he grows up with diabetes. Without supporting his development, increasing his knowledge, and teaching him the decision-making skills he will need to successfully manage his diabetes, Michael will one day be on his own and his health may suffer. He may be more dependent on his parents for guidance and direction regarding basic care issues that he could have developed for himself over time.

Sam has been exposed to increasing responsibility for self-care. She has also been involved in making decisions regarding treatment options and has seen first hand how her parents and the physicians, and her Mom and the cafeteria staff work to resolve things. Although she may feel powerless with the cafeteria staff right now, Sam has been given a voice to express her needs regarding her treatment and with the continued support and guidance from her parents, she will develop the self-care maintenance, monitoring and management skills required for optimal outcomes.

SUMMARY

For self-care to be successful, all 3 components, self-care maintenance, self-care monitoring, and self-care management, must be developed with increasing capacity for health care autonomy. Children with chronic health conditions may learn basic maintenance skills, and seem competent, but unless attention is paid to teaching them monitoring and management, as they mature and expectations are placed on them, they will not be successful. Paying attention to the components of self-care, as well as the family management style and the developmental abilities of the child, will help nurses assess the care status and create a plan to assist the child and family with the care transitions.

Further research is needed on incorporating health care autonomy, self-care, and family management. Studies aimed at testing interventions to improve child health outcomes throughout adolescence and into young adulthood may assist children and families as they progress through this challenging transition.

RECOMMENDATIONS FOR THE FAMILY

- When communicating with a partner and other family members, remember the importance of helping the child to become able to take care of himself/herself over time and planning to do so.

- When communicating with the child, remember to support self-reliance/self-competence. Increase the use of guidance and monitoring as opposed to authoritative parenting.
  - Retain appropriate parental agency throughout school-aged years into adolescence; this allows for the development of health care autonomy but enables safety and adherence for the child.
  - Develop skills in parental monitoring to encourage adherence and safety, especially during self-care transitions; that is, continue monitoring and involvement throughout the school-aged years into adolescence even when the child seems able to perform basic skills independently because re-involvement during adolescence is difficult.

RECOMMENDATIONS FOR THE PROVIDER

Interventions to develop self-care need to consider

- Assessing child readiness for self-care including developmental stage, self-reliance, physical, cognitive, and psychosocial ability, and the parent-child relationship
- Assessing agency: who is driving the condition management (parents, shared, or child) and determination of appropriateness based on the child's development
- Teaching skills for parental monitoring that are developmentally appropriate
- Assisting the family and child with culturally appropriate interventions to transition to self-care, including responsibilities for self-care maintenance (behaviors), self-care monitoring (body listening), and self-care management (evaluation)

REFERENCES

1. Chronic diseases: the power to prevent, the call to control. At a glance 2009. Available at: http://www.cdc.gov/chronicdisease/resource/publications/AAG/chronic.htm. Accessed August 20, 2012.
2. Hagan JF, Shaw JS, Duncan PM. Bright futures: guidelines for health supervision of infants, children, and adolescents. 3rd edition. Elk Grove Village (IL): American Academy of Pediatrics; 2008.
3. Gortmaker SL, Sappenfield W. Chronic childhood disorders - prevalence and impact. Pediatr Clin North Am 1984;31(1):3–18.
4. Cohen E, Kuo DZ, Agrawal R, et al. Children with medical complexity: an emerging population for clinical and research initiatives. Pediatrics 2011;127(3):529–38.
5. American Academy of Pediatrics, American Academy of Family Physicians, American College of Physicians, Transitions Clinical Report Authoring Group. Supporting the health care transition from adolescence to adulthood in the medical home. Pediatrics 2011;128(1):182–200.
6. Newacheck PW, Stein RE, Walker DK, et al. Monitoring and evaluating managed care for children with chronic illnesses and disabilities. Pediatrics 1996;98(5):952–8.
7. Noom MJ, Dekovic M, Meeus W. Conceptual analysis and measurement of adolescent autonomy. J Youth Adolesc 2001;30(5):577–95.
8. Smetana JG, Campione-Barr N, Daddis C. Longitudinal development of family decision making: defining healthy behavioral autonomy for middle-class African American adolescents. Child Dev 2004;75(5):1418–34.
9. Wray-Lake L, Crouter AC, McHale SM. Developmental patterns in decision-making autonomy across middle childhood and adolescence: European American parents' perspectives. Child Dev 2010;81(2):636–51.

10. Schwartz LA, Tuchman LK, Hobbie WL, et al. A social-ecological model of readiness for transition to adult-oriented care for adolescents and young adults with chronic health conditions. Child Care Health Dev 2011;37(6):883–95.
11. Knafl KA, Deatrick JA, Havill NL. Continued development of the family management style framework. J Fam Nurs 2012;18(1):11–34.
12. Cadman D, Boyle M, Szatmari P, et al. Chronic illness, disability, and mental and social wellbeing: findings of the Ontario child health study. Pediatrics 1987;79(5): 805.
13. Suris JC, Michaud PA, Viner R. The adolescent with a chronic condition. Part I: developmental issues. Arch Dis Child 2004;89(10):938–42.
14. Wollenhaupt J, Rodgers B, Sawin KJ. Family management of a chronic health condition. J Fam Nurs 2012;18(1):65–90.
15. Riegel B, Jaarsma T, Stromberg A. A middle-range theory of self-care of chronic illness. ANS Adv Nurs Sci 2012;35(3):194–204.
16. Weissberg-Benchell J, Goodman SS, Lomaglio JA, et al. The use of continuous subcutaneous insulin infusion (CSII): parental and professional perceptions of self-care mastery and autonomy in children and adolescents. J Pediatr Psychol 2007;32(10):1196–202.
17. Pradel FG, Hartzema AG, Bush PJ. Asthma self-management: the perspective of children. Patient Educ Couns 2001;45(3):199–209.
18. Fiese BH, Everhart RS. Medical adherence and childhood chronic illness: family daily management skills and emotional climate as emerging contributors. Curr Opin Pediatr 2006;18(5):551–7.
19. Helgeson VS, Novak SA. Illness centrality and well-being among male and female early adolescents with diabetes. J Pediatr Psychol 2007;32(3):260–72.
20. Beacham B. Developing autonomy: implications for children with chronic health conditions. Philadelphia: University of Pennsylvania; 2011.
21. Coatsworth JD, Conroy DE. The effects of autonomy-supportive coaching, need satisfaction, and self-perceptions on initiative and identity in youth swimmers. Dev Psychol 2009;45(2):320–8.
22. Eccles JS, Early D, Frasier K, et al. The relation of connection, regulation, and support for autonomy to adolescents' functioning. J Adolesc Res 1997;12(2): 263–86.
23. Vansteenkiste M, Simons J, Lens W, et al. Examining the motivational impact of intrinsic versus extrinsic goal framing and autonomy-supportive versus internally controlling communication style on early adolescents' academic achievement. Child Dev 2005;76(2):483–501.
24. Dashiff CJ, Weaver M. Development and testing of a scale to measure separation anxiety of parents of adolescents. J Nurs Meas 2008;16(1):61–80.
25. Butner J, Berg CA, Osborn P, et al. Parent-adolescent discrepancies in adolescents' competence and the balance of adolescent autonomy and adolescent and parent well-being in the context of Type 1 diabetes. Dev Psychol 2009; 45(3):835–49.
26. Weinger K, O'Donnell KA, Ritholz MD. Adolescent views of diabetes-related parent conflict and support: a focus group analysis. J Adolesc Health 2001; 29(5):330–6.
27. Wiebe DJ, Berg CA, Korbel C, et al. Children's appraisals of maternal involvement in coping with diabetes: enhancing our understanding of adherence, metabolic control, and quality of life across adolescence. J Pediatr Psychol 2005;30(2): 167–78.

Promoting Normal Development and Self-Efficacy in School-Age Children Managing Chronic Conditions

Kristyn L. Mickley, BSN, RN[a,b,*], Patricia V. Burkhart, PhD, RN[a],
April N. Sigler, BA[c]

KEYWORDS

- Chronic illness • Self-efficacy • Self-management • Normal development

KEY POINTS

- Chronic conditions may affect school-age children not only physically but also emotionally and developmentally.
- Self-management behaviors are the necessary skills and activities to control symptoms of a chronic condition.
- Behavioral strategies that promote self-management of chronic conditions, including those that encourage self-efficacy, the self-belief that a person can effectively perform necessary skills, are essential to promoting children's skills in disease management, and can contribute positively to children's normal development.

INTRODUCTION

Chronic conditions are becoming more prevalent in the United States, affecting 10 to 20 million children and adolescents.[1] These long-term conditions may affect school-age children emotionally, physically, and developmentally. The symptoms can be challenging for the children, but the management and treatment are additional burdens. Normal developmental patterns may be interrupted with a diagnosis of a chronic illness. However, if children learn to effectively self-manage their disease, the focus can be redirected to promote normal development. This article reviews the theoretical and empirical literature to describe chronic illnesses and their impact on the development of school-age children. Behavioral strategies supporting

a 202 College of Nursing, University of Kentucky, 751 Rose Street, Lexington, KY 40536-0232, USA; b Pediatric Intensive Care Unit, Kentucky Children's Hospital, Lexington, KY 40536-0232, USA; c School Psychology, College of Education, University of Kentucky, 751 Rose Street, Lexington, KY 40536-0232, USA
* Corresponding author. 202 College of Nursing, University of Kentucky, 751 Rose Street, Lexington, KY 40536-0232.
E-mail address: klmick2@uky.edu

self-management skills, including those that promote self-efficacy, when combined with education can also promote appropriate childhood development. Self-efficacy is defined as the self-belief that one can effectively perform necessary skills. Identifying and implementing effective strategies to promote self-efficacy in children managing a chronic condition may contribute to children's health and well-being.

COMMON CHILDHOOD CHRONIC CONDITIONS AND MANAGEMENT

According to the World Health Organization, chronic diseases are those that have a lengthy duration (ie, longer than 3 months) and usually develop slowly.[2] Childhood chronic illnesses present challenges to families, with complex treatment regimens and tasks that interfere with daily activities. Common childhood illnesses in school-age children such as asthma, seizure disorders, diabetes, and cystic fibrosis, and their management, are discussed here.

Asthma

Asthma is a chronic lung disorder affecting 7 million children in the United States.[3] With this disease there is narrowing of the airways caused by inflammation and mucus production, resulting in airway obstruction. Asthma is characterized by coughing, wheezing, difficulty in breathing, and tightness in the chest.[4] It is diagnosed by the presenting symptoms and spirometric evaluation of how fast air can be exhaled from the lungs.[4] Asthma exacerbations, known as asthma attacks, result from an insult or irritation to the airways, referred to as triggers. Some of the more common asthma triggers include respiratory infections and environmental elements, such as pollution, mold, dust mites, and tobacco smoke.[4] Asthma is controllable if triggers are avoided and appropriate medications to control inflammation are taken. Long-term medications to help prevent attacks and quick-relief medicines to help during attack are available.[4] An asthma action (management) plan should be developed with the health care provider to guide daily treatment for long-term symptom control.[5]

Seizure Disorders

Seizure disorders are prevalent in 2 million people in the United States, and most are diagnosed in children younger than 2 years.[6] A seizure disorder is a chronic neurologic condition with reoccurring abnormal electrical activity in the brain leading to involuntary changes in behavior, motor function, perception, or awareness,[7] which can vary from short episodes of unconsciousness to convulsions.[7] To manage seizures, health care providers determine the type of seizure and underlying condition that may have caused the seizures. Through a combination of medical history, neurologic examinations, electroencephalograms, computed tomography scan of the brain, or even magnetic resonance imaging of the brain, a specific diagnosis is made.[8] Based on the evaluation, antiseizure medications are selected to control the particular type of seizures. Once medication therapy is initiated, monitoring is required to assess whether adjustments in the medications are needed. Another treatment option is surgery, especially when the area of the brain where a seizure arises can be specifically identified. A diet high in fat and low in carbohydrates with restricted calories, called a ketogenic diet, is effective in some patients with seizures.[8] Regardless of the type of seizure, a daily regimen of medication and symptom monitoring is required.

Diabetes

Type 1 diabetes is newly diagnosed in more than 15,600 youth each year.[9] For children younger than 10 years, new cases were diagnosed in 19.7 per 100,000 children each year for type 1 diabetes,[9] whereas for those 10 years and older there were 18.6 cases per 100,000.[9] Type 1 diabetes is a disease affecting the body's metabolism of glucose. The food ingested is converted to glucose, which is used for energy. The pancreas secretes the hormone insulin, which helps glucose to enter the cells to produce energy. If the body cannot make enough insulin (type 1 diabetes) or is not able to use the insulin effectively (type 2 diabetes), excess glucose builds up in the body.[10] Excess blood sugar over the long term can cause complications, such as "heart disease, blindness, kidney failure, and lower extremity amputations".[10(p1)] Short-term symptoms include "frequent urination, excessive thirst, unexplained weight loss, extreme hunger, sudden vision changes, tingling or numbness in hands or feet, feeling very tired much of the time, very dry skin, sores that are slow to heal, [and] more infections than usual".[10(p1)]

To treat the symptoms of type 1 diabetes, patients administer insulin based on the amount of food intake and expenditure of energy with daily lifestyle. Close monitoring of blood glucose levels is critical. Along with insulin, treatment regimens are supplemented with a healthy diet and physical activity. It is also important for patients with type 2 diabetes to eat well, be active, and monitor their blood glucose levels on a regular basis. Oral medication is the most common early treatment for type 2 diabetes. It is important to ensure that an individual's blood glucose level never becomes too low or too high at any point in time. Glucose control should be monitored by the patient and reviewed with a health care provider at each health care encounter.[10]

Cystic Fibrosis

Cystic fibrosis (CF) is a progressive genetic disease of the body's mucus glands that affects 30,000 people in the United States.[11] Approximately 2500 infants are born each year with CF.[11] The respiratory system and digestive system are primary targets of this disease, as well as the sweat glands and the reproductive system. Abnormal glands produce or secrete excess sweat and mucus. CF patients lose large amounts of salt, creating an imbalance of minerals in their body. Mucus production is also thick, and accumulates in the intestine and lungs. Because of these impairments, nutritional deficiency can occur resulting in poor growth. Frequent respiratory infections are common, which can eventually cause permanent and even fatal lung damage.[11]

CF treatment is focused on controlling the symptoms to delay the progression of the disease and improve the quality of life. The recommended daily therapy is individualized and symptom specific. To manage respiratory involvement and reduction of mucus blockage, medications are supplemented with physical therapy. Chest physiotherapy to promote bronchial drainage is done by placing the patient in various positions and percussing the chest and back to dislodge and remove mucus.[11] This process is repeated on a daily basis. Usually parents perform this process for younger children, but as children grow older they can learn to do it on their own. Aerosolized and inhaled agents, such as bronchodilators, mucolytics, and decongestants, are common medications prescribed. Antibiotic therapy is used for clearing the thick mucus from the lungs and to treat lung infections. To help with digestive-system problems, a diet with low fat, high protein, and high calories, supplemented with pancreatic enzymes, is necessary. Daily supplements of vitamins A, D, E, and K help with the deficiency. In the incidence of an obstruction, enemas and mucolytics are used. The recommended treatment regimen is required on a daily basis.[11]

DEVELOPMENTAL ASPECTS OF THE SCHOOL-AGE CHILD

In 1962 Jean Piaget explained that 7- to 11-year-old children are in the cognitive phase of concrete operations.[12] According to this stage, school-age children can think rationally in varied situations. Piaget also discusses how children interact with objects. School-agers should be able to compare objects based on coinciding characteristics and incongruities. Objects are placed in a serializing format by either size, weight, or other classifications. Problem-solving skills begin around age 7 years.[12]

Moral realism is also developing in the school-age child, with emphasis on rules and responsibility. Assuming responsibility means being a good person by obeying the rules.[12] For children, obeying the rules simply means doing what is asked of them no matter the discernment. In the end, children will discover their own personal moral rules, usually based on upbringing.[12]

Psychosocial aspects of school-age children, outlined by Erikson[13] in 1950, involve developing a sense of industry. A sense of industry is achieved by having successful outcomes and accomplishments. The work ethic becomes more concentrated as the child perseveres in varied situations. The main focus for children is competition among peers as they become reassured of their abilities. The relationship children have with their friends is more important than a family-focused life. Children are ready to tackle adult tasks and apply them to their world. A sense of worth and success comes from feeling part of a peer group and accomplishing tasks. Parents and schools offer role models children can imitate.[13]

On the other hand, if children do not achieve the same level as their peers or do not find success in the world, they develop a sense of inferiority. Failing to meet their parents' or personal expectations may also lead to this sense of inadequacy. Children at this age tend to find their worth in success, so if they consistently lose in competitions they may withdraw and become isolated. If this continues, the children's actual capabilities are at risk.[13]

EFFECTS OF CHRONIC ILLNESS ON DEVELOPMENT OF THE SCHOOL-AGE CHILD

When facing chronic illness, children may have diminished opportunities for peer interaction and irregular school attendance. If children constantly have to interrupt their activities to take medication or monitor symptoms, they miss activities and may lose interest in interacting with other children. Sometimes symptom exacerbations can cause the child to be too sick to attend school, resulting in time away from peers and interruption of their education.[14]

Children want to master skills and engage in social interactions. Because children with chronic illnesses may have decreased interactions with peers, normal skill development can lag. Children with a chronic illness may also feel different to their peers, preventing them from establishing social networks. In turn this can hinder self-esteem and the children's sense of mastery, leading to underachievement.[14]

Medication management may be difficult when the time comes for the child to attend school. At home, it can be very easy for the parent to lend assistance, but when it comes to managing and administering medication at school, children need to be assessed to determine whether they need assistance. In a study examining the experiences of children 5 to 18 years old with chronic conditions and their parents, 6 main areas of medication-related issues at school were identified.[15] If children only used the medication occasionally or when needed, they had more limited access to it. Many children did not believe they had a private place to take their medication, and often felt embarrassed. A third problem was the impact of adverse effects of the medications, which led to children not taking their medications while at school, thus affecting their treatment. Fourth, the chronic illness and its treatment were barriers to the children's participation in extracurricular activities and school trips. For some children, the need for medication could result in exclusion from school trips. Attitudes of peers are a fifth barrier to the use of medicines in school. Finally, the support in school was not as strong as desired. Many parents did not get the support they desired for their child until they exerted pressure on the teacher or administration. Management issues for children with chronic conditions and their parents were identified not only in their lives at home but also at school.[15]

It is also important to understand the unique challenges parents face when managing their child's chronic illness. A qualitative study explored the relationship of 18 youth (8–19 years old) and their parents who were interviewed about management of the child's health-related behaviors.[16] Most parents monitored whether their children took their medicine or did their treatment by using tracking materials for treatment adherence. Examples were assessing whether the inhalers were used, test strips used for glucose monitoring, or counting the number of tablets.[16] Both the parent and the child reported that nagging and recurrent reminders regarding treatment were common. Some parents monitored treatment adherence by requiring the child to perform the behavior in their presence. Many parents sought control by impeding activities that might exacerbate the illness, or providing time restraints on children's activities to support regimen adherence. In summary, the parents felt they had an obligation to carefully monitor their child's treatment but also realized a balance was necessary for the child's normal development.[16] Parents struggled to facilitate adherence that created stress for themselves and their children. The parents first wanted their children to attest they could handle the responsibility. Of course, children did not always respond to the parents' pleas appropriately. Some children viewed their parents' supervision as extreme and annoying, leading some children to attempt to prove themselves to their parents or find ways to avoid the required behaviors.[16]

An adult and child version of an Asthma Responsibility Interview was developed to evaluate perceptions of responsibility for asthma management for families of inner-city children (N = 789), aged 6 to 9 years.[17] The results indicated that the degree of responsibility of the child tended to increase with age; however, the parent's (or caregiver's) responsibility remained consistent. Because the degree of responsibility was increasing for the child, the parents felt the need to monitor and supervise more, not less, closely. These findings suggest that health care providers need a clear understanding of responsibility for treatment management in the family and whether the responsibility for the child's self-management is age appropriate.[17]

Self-Management

Self-management is defined as the skills and activities necessary to control symptoms of a chronic condition.[18] Chronic conditions require daily management that can be time consuming. Everyday lifestyles are altered but can be managed by the application of effective models to embrace positive self-management behaviors. It is important to appropriately define key components of self-management to increase adherence. For the individual diagnosed with chronic illness, self-management focuses on identifying specific knowledge, skills, and activities related to the illness, activating essential resources, and learning to live with a chronic illness.[19] Education about the disease and the skills to manage symptoms are required. Activating resources not only includes accessing community resources but also soliciting the families to form support groups as appropriate. Living with chronic illness includes the transition and adjustment of tasks and skills required as part of the individual's lifestyle. Emotions are an important aspect of self-management. Factors that interfere with self-management include socioeconomic status and culture, complexity of the treatment regimen, and relationship with the health care provider.[19] The family's motivation and belief that they can handle the situation also contributes to effective self-management.

Self-Efficacy

An alternative to parental nagging is to harness school-age children's desire to be industrious; that is, children's need to accomplish tasks and be reassured of their abilities. This task can be accomplished by teaching the children self-management strategies incrementally and reinforcing their small successes. The link between self-efficacy and the ability to self-manage chronic illness is important.

Self-efficacy is the belief in one's ability to perform certain actions.[20] Self-efficacy is influential in a variety of human actions, including self-management. Our beliefs about what we are capable of doing strongly influence our choices and decisions, as well as our effort and persistence.[21] Low self-efficacy, or perceived deficiencies, can cause people to imagine tasks to be far more difficult than they actually are.[21] The result may be avoidance of difficult tasks. For children with a chronic illness, low self-efficacy could mean that they envision their daily self-management tasks to be more than they can adequately handle.

The relationship between self-efficacy and asthma self-management was examined in a study of 81 African American children aged 7 to 12 years.[22] The researcher administered 2 instruments: the Asthma Inventory for Children (AIC), which measures self-management behaviors, and the Asthma Belief Survey (ABS), which measures self-efficacy. A significant positive correlation was found between self-management behaviors and self-efficacy ($r = 0.529$, $P<.01$). Children who scored high on the self-efficacy scale, reporting they believed they could manage their asthma well, had increased scores on the asthma self-management scale, meaning that the children who reported using more self-management behaviors to control their asthma believed they could do so effectively. Children with lower self-efficacy scores reported less frequent use of self-management strategies.[22] These findings are consistent with those of previous research that self-efficacy correlates with illness-management behaviors in children.[23] Children's belief that they are able to manage their illness allows them to complete tasks. When they successfully complete tasks, they build a sense of industry.[13]

Self-efficacy was also found to be strongly associated with children making healthy food choices. For example, children with diabetes were more likely to choose healthy foods if they had higher self-efficacy.[24] Low self-efficacy was associated with increased worry and a higher need for psychosocial care in 173 children (9–14 years) with seizure disorders.[25]

Increased self-efficacy can be beneficial to children's healthy development not only in terms of treatment management but also by building their confidence for participation in everyday activities. Asthma self-efficacy beliefs and participation in physical activity was examined in 172 adolescent females (14–18 years old) from a private inner-city high school.[26] Twenty-two percent of the participants had previously been diagnosed with asthma. An additional 15% of the girls reported breathing difficulties. The researchers administered a lung health questionnaire that included demographic questions, smoking practices, physical factors, and asthma management and self-regulation skills. The participants were also administered a lung self-efficacy scale that asked the girls to report confidence in their ability to engage in 25 specific physical activities without experiencing breathing problems. The subjects were given a test of physical fitness and an activity log, in which the girls recorded time spent participating in physical activity.[26] The results suggested that the asthmatic girls were less physically fit, reported lower self-efficacy in terms of their lung functioning during physical activity, and participated in physical activity less often than the nonasthmatic girls. Lung self-efficacy perception was positively correlated with participation in physical activity. Self-efficacy was the most predictive of activity levels. Few girls reported using self-management strategies to prevent or control their asthma attacks. High levels of symptoms were reported, including 87% of the girls reporting that asthma symptoms were present "often" or "most of the time." The researchers concluded that increasing feelings of self-efficacy, by effective use of asthma self-management behaviors, would decrease the severity and frequency of symptoms. Children are less likely to have physical activity restrictions if they feel confident in their ability to implement self-management methods to prevent asthma symptoms.[26] These findings were consistent with previous studies that indicated a positive correlation between self-efficacy and health status, and a negative correlation between self-efficacy and asthma symptoms.[27]

Although self-efficacy seems to play a major role in a child's self-management, many parents may not feel ready to transfer all of the responsibility to their child immediately. The following models are examples of effective ways to transfer responsibility.

The developmental model focuses on normal childhood development. Disease management is transferred from the parent to the child as the child matures. Parents need to not only understand how to manage the child's illness but also be cognizant of the developmental milestones when transferring illness care to the child.[28]

In the leadership model, parents manage all the direct care when the child is first diagnosed.[28] The care is given over to the child once the child develops experience and skill in the management of the disease. The parent is considered the "manager" and the child the "provider" of care. The parent should still be ready to intervene at any time necessary. When the parent feels ready, the parent becomes the "supervisor." This changeover should happen when the child feels even more comfortable with managing the disease. If these steps are followed properly and not rushed, the parent can ultimately become the "consultant." This model can be very successful, especially if incorporated with the developmental model.[28]

Changing the foci directs families to keep the focus on the child's normal development during times of wellness, relegating condition-specific needs to the background of the child's life unless exacerbations occur.[28] An example is for a child with asthma to be encouraged to participate in gym class by premedicating before exercise. An individualized asthma action plan directs the actions to be taken if symptom exacerbation occurs during an activity. This plan will help the child manage the disease, but then put it back out of focus once the symptoms are managed. Planning ahead and anticipation are important in normalizing the child's life.[28]

IMPLICATIONS FOR CLINICAL PRACTICE AND RESEARCH

Chronic illness poses unique challenges for children. Regardless of the type of chronic condition, long-term management is required, and the child's normal developmental milestones must be considered. Education and developmentally appropriate self-management strategies, tailored to the particular needs of the child and family, are needed.

The current standard of care for children diagnosed with chronic conditions is to educate the child and family about the disease and the importance of adhering to the recommended treatment. However, adherence to self-management remains low.[29] Education alone is not sufficient to ensure adherence.[29] Combining education with behavioral strategies improves treatment adherence.[30] The contingency management model, based on cognitive social learning theory, is a behavioral model that shows promise for promoting the adherence to recommended self-management behaviors.[31] Contingency management includes behaviors such as self-monitoring, cueing, tailoring, reinforcing, and contracting. Such behaviors are also appropriate to the normal development of school-age children.[31]

Self-monitoring consists of tracking symptoms to ensure that treatment goals are being achieved. Cueing is a visual reminder, such as sticky note, to remember to take medication. Tailoring connects the treatment regimen to the child's daily routine. Reinforcing and rewarding expected behaviors establish a pattern for repeating such behaviors. A contract between the parent, child, and health care provider outlines the expected behavior and the reward. Contracts are well received by school-age children, who appreciate knowing the rules.[31]

Using a multistrategy approach, such as contingency management that supports self-efficacy, has the potential to change clinical practice with school-age children diagnosed with a chronic condition, because it is more likely than education alone to promote adherence.[29] By combining education with the contingency management model, children are more likely to successfully self-manage their disease.[30] Future research is needed to test the efficacy of the models used in teaching self-management skills to school-age children with various chronic conditions, such as those discussed here.

Health care providers are in a position to develop protocols, based on empirical evidence, which support parent and child partnerships in the management of chronic conditions. Children's illnesses do not have to be interferences in children's lives; rather, they can be opportunities to encourage age-appropriate responsibility, with a focus on successful achievements. This concept includes school-age children's belief that they can effectively manage chronic symptoms.

SUMMARY

How children and their parents perceive the management of chronic disease illustrates the critical need for an evidence-based protocol whereby health care providers can educate parents and their children on how to deal with the management of chronic illness. To prevent delays in normal childhood development, treatment needs to be redirected to promote and advance children's development. Further research is needed to test strategies for using a multistrategy behavioral model. The combination of the self-efficacy model and the contingency management model is an example of a multistrategy approach that shows promise for success.

Health care professionals have the opportunity to teach behaviors to children and families that not only manage symptoms but also promote a normal, healthy life. Protocols need to be developed and used by health care providers to assist families in helping children to manage their condition at home. Evidence-based protocols that incorporate effective self-management strategies, promote self-efficacy, and support normal childhood development will contribute to successful health outcomes for children and their families.

ACKNOWLEDGMENTS

As first author, I (K.L.Mickley) would like to thank my mentor, Dr Patricia Burkhart, for her continuing support of my education, research, and career goals and for her contributions to the development of this article. I would also like to thank the coauthor, April Sigler, for her contributions.

REFERENCES

1. American Academy of Pediatrics. Chronic conditions. 2011. Available at: http://www. healthychildren.org/English/health-issues/conditions/chronic/Pages/default.aspx? nfstatus=401&nftoken=00000000-0000-0000-0000-000000000000&nfstatus description=ERROR%3a+No+local+token&nfstatus=401&nftoken=00000000-0000-0000-0000-000000000000&nfstatusdescription=ERROR%3a+No+local+ token. Accessed September 23, 2012.
2. World Health Organization. Chronic diseases. 2011. Available at: http://www.who. int/topics/chronic_diseases/en/. Accessed June 17, 2012.
3. Centers for Disease Control and Prevention. Asthma. 2012. Available at: http:// www.cdc.gov/nchs/fastats/asthma.htm. Accessed June 17, 2012.
4. Centers for Disease Control and Prevention. Asthma: basic information. 2012. Available at: http://www.cdc.gov/asthma/faqs.htm. Accessed June 17, 2012.
5. Centers for Disease Control and Prevention. Asthma: asthma action plan. 2012. Available at: http://www.cdc.gov/asthma/actionplan.html. Accessed June 17, 2012.
6. Centers for Disease Control and Prevention. Announcements: national epilepsy awareness month—November 2011. 2011. Available at: http://www.cdc.gov/ mmwr/preview/mmwrhtml/mm6043a5.htm?s_cid=mm6043a5_w. Accessed June 17, 2012.
7. Center for Disease Control and Prevention. Targeting epilepsy. 2011. Available at: http://www.cdc.gov/chronicdisease/resources/publications/AAG/epilepsy.htm. Accessed June 17, 2012.
8. Center for Disease Control and Prevention. Epilepsy: frequently asked questions. 2010. Available at: http://www.cdc.gov/epilepsy/basics/faqs.htm#7. Accessed August 17, 2012.
9. Centers for Disease Control and Prevention. New cases of diagnosed diabetes among people younger than 20 years of age, United States, 2002-2005. 2011. Available at: http://www.cdc.gov/diabetes/pubs/estimates11.htm#1. Accessed June 17, 2012.
10. Centers for Disease Control and Prevention. Basics about diabetes. 2012. Available at: http://www.cdc.gov/diabetes/consumer/learn.htm. Accessed June 17, 2012.
11. Centers for Disease Control and Prevention. Facts about cystic fibrosis. 1995. Available at: http://www.cdc.gov/excite/ScienceAmbassador/ambassador_pgm/ lessonplans/high_school/Am%20I%20a%20Carrier%20for%20Cystic%20Fibrosis/ Cystic_Fibrosis_Fact_Sheet.pdf. Accessed June 17, 2012.
12. Piaget J, Inhelder B. The psychology of the child. New York: Basic Books, Inc.; 1969. p. 93–106, 126.
13. Erikson EH. Childhood and society. New York: Norton & Company, Inc.; 1950. p. 258–61.
14. Yoos L. Chronic childhood illnesses: developmental issues. Pediatr Nurs 1987; 13:25–8.
15. Smith F, Taylor K, Newbould J, et al. Medicines for chronic illness at school: experiences and concerns of young people and their parents. J Clin Pharm Ther 2008; 33:537–44.
16. Hafetz J, Miller V. Child and parent perceptions of monitoring in chronic illness management: a qualitative study. Child Care Health Dev 2010;36:655–62.

17. Wade S, Islam S, Holden G, et al. Division of responsibility for asthma management tasks between caregivers and children in the inner city. J Dev Behav Pediatr 1999;20:93–8.

18. Centers for Disease Control and Prevention. Glossary terms: self-management. 2011. Available at: http://www.cdc.gov/workplacehealthpromotion/glossary/. Accessed August 24, 2012.

19. Schulman-Green D, Jaser S, Martin F, et al. Processes of self-management in chronic illness. J Nurs Scholarsh 2012;44:136.

20. Bandura A. Self-efficacy: the exercise of control. New York: H. Freeman and Company; 1997. p. 21.

21. Thoresen C, Kirmil-Gray K. Self-management psychology and the treatment of childhood asthma. J Allergy Clin Immunol 1983;72:596–606.

22. Kaul T. Helping African American children self-manage asthma: the importance of self-efficacy. J Sch Health 2011;81:29–33.

23. Clark N, Rosenstock I, Hassan H, et al. The effect of health beliefs and feelings of self efficacy on self- management behavior of children with a chronic disease. Patient Educ Counsel 1988;11:131–9.

24. Parcel G, Edmundson E, Perry C, et al. Measurement of self-efficacy for diet-related behaviors among elementary school children. J Sch Health 1995;65:23–7.

25. Austin J, Dunn D, Perkins S, et al. Youth with epilepsy: development of a model of children's attitudes toward their condition. Child Health Care 2006;35:123–40.

26. Kitsantas A, Zimmerman B. Self-efficacy, activity participation, and physical fitness of asthmatic and nonasthmatic adolescent girls. J Asthma 2000;37: 163–74.

27. Bursch B, Schwankovsky L, Gilbert J, et al. Construction and validation of four childhood asthma self-management scales: parent barriers, child and parent self-efficacy, and parent belief in treatment efficacy. J Asthma 1999;36:115–28.

28. Kieckhefer GM, Trahms CM. Supporting development of children with chronic conditions: From compliance toward shared management. Pediatr Nurs 2000; 26:354–63, 380–1.

29. Burkhart P, Dunbar-Jacob J. Adherence research in the pediatric and adolescent populations: a decade in review. In: Hayman L, Mahon M, Turner R, editors. New York (NY): Springer; Chronic illness in children: an evidence-based approach. vol. 1. 2002. p. 199–229.

30. Burkhart P, Rayens M, Oakley M, et al. Testing an intervention to promote children's adherence to asthma self-management. J Nurs Scholarsh 2007;39: 133–40.

31. Burkhart P, Oakley M, Mickley K. Self-management for school-age children with asthma. Curr Pediatr Rev 2012;8:45–50.

Developmental Mastery of Diabetes-Related Tasks in Children

Leslie K. Scott, PhD, PNP-BC, CDE

KEYWORDS

- Diabetes in children • Self-management in children • Task mastery
- Child development in diabetes

KEY POINTS

- Poor management can have a negative impact on a child's growth and development.
- Having an understanding of child development and cognitive development ensures adequate expectations of self-care skill acquisition.
- Numerous steps can be taken to assist the child with diabetes in developmentally appropriate transition of self-care skills.

Diabetes is the second most common chronic condition affecting children. It is estimated that 15,000 children are diagnosed with type 1 diabetes and 3700 are diagnosed with type 2 annually.[1] Type 1 diabetes remains the most common form of diabetes seen in children. Type 1 diabetes is an autoimmune disease in which the insulin-producing β cells of the pancreas are destroyed.[2] As a result, individuals with type 1 diabetes require insulin to sustain life. The pathophysiology of type 2 diabetes is multifactorial and may require insulin therapy to meet glycemic management goals.[2] Over the past 15 years, disease management of diabetes in children has changed significantly. Regimens have developed from management regimens aimed at minimizing hypoglycemia and diabetic ketoacidosis to a more individualized approach aimed at mimicking normal glucose metabolic response to carbohydrate (CHO) intake and energy expenditure. The standard of care for children with diabetes (type 1 diabetes), regardless of their age at onset, has become one that includes multiple daily insulin dosing (vial/syringe, pen device, insulin pump), frequent blood glucose monitoring, CHO counting, and daily activity. Type 2 diabetes management in children is no less intrusive to lifestyle adjustments than type 1 diabetes.[3] Additional childhood diabetes management includes acquiring skills to manage fluctuations in

Disclosures: No disclosures or 'conflicts of interest'.
College of Nursing, University of Kentucky, 425A College of Nursing Building, 801 Rose Street, Lexington, KY 40536, USA
E-mail address: lkscot0@uky.edu

Nurs Clin N Am 48 (2013) 329–342
http://dx.doi.org/10.1016/j.cnur.2013.01.015
0029-6465/13/$ – see front matter © 2013 Elsevier Inc. All rights reserved.

nursing.theclinics.com

daily schedule, medication needs, dietary patterns, and issues during illness to foster normal growth and development during childhood.

DIABETES MANAGEMENT IN CHILDREN

The goal of managing diabetes in childhood is to assist the child in becoming a physically healthy and emotionally mature adult, free from complications associated with diabetes.[3] Gradual achievement of self-care independence occurs as developmental changes evolve during childhood. Inappropriate expectations related to self-care competence may lead to impaired diabetes control.[4]

Although current management guidelines and glycemic goals for controlling diabetes emphasize the need to maintain near-normal glucose control, special considerations need to be taken into account regarding management in children, particularly in regards to safety and risk of hypoglycemia (**Table 1**).[5] Poor management can have a negative impact on a child's growth and development. Many issues associated with diabetes management in children are a direct result of a child's developmental age and cognitive development skill level. It is important for parents, health professionals, and others caring for the child with diabetes to have an understanding of child development and cognitive development in order to ensure adequate expectations of self-care skill acquisition and the appropriate transition of self-care skills.

SKILLS NEEDED TO MASTER DIABETES-RELATED TASKS

Children need to acquire various cognitive, motor, and psychosocial skills to master the numerous tasks associated with diabetes self-care. The primary self-care skills

Table 1
Glycemic goals for children with diabetes

Plasma Blood Glucose Goals (mg/dL) for Children with Diabetes by Age				
Age (y)	Before Meals	Bedtime/Overnight	A1c (%)	Rationale
0–5	100–180	110–200	<8.5	Vulnerability to hypoglycemia Insulin sensitivity Unpredictability in dietary intake and physical activity A lower goal (<8%) is reasonable if it can be achieved without excessive hypoglycemia
6–12	90–180	100–180	<8	Vulnerability to hypoglycemia A lower goal (<7.5%) is reasonable if it can be achieved without excessive hypoglycemia
13–18	90–130	90–150	<7.5	A lower goal (<7%) is reasonable if it can be achieved without excessive hypoglycemia

Key Concepts in Setting Glycemic Goals
Goals should be individualized
Blood glucose goals should be modified in children with frequent hypoglycemia or hypoglycemia unawareness
Consider measuring postprandial blood glucose values when there is a discrepancy between blood glucose values and A1c levels or to help assess glycemic excursions in those on basal/bolus therapy.

Data from American Diabetes Association. Standards of medical care in diabetes–2012 position statement. Diabetes Care 2012;35(Suppl 1):S11–6.

inherent to diabetes management in children include blood glucose monitoring, medication administration (insulin or oral agents), CHO intake (consistent CHO intake vs CHO counting), hypoglycemia/hyperglycemia detection and management, emergency management, and the impact of physical activity on insulin sensitivity and resistance.[5] Psychosocial issues and poor glycemic control may arise if children with diabetes lack any of these cognitive, motor, or psychosocial skills before the transition of these self-care tasks.[4]

TRANSITION OF CARE IN CHILDREN

Ideally, the transition of diabetes-related, self-care skills to children should take into consideration the parent's knowledge of their child's abilities as well as health care providers drawing on knowledge and experience with diabetes management in children and developmental capabilities of children at various ages.[4] As diabetes management regimens and integration of technology into self-care skills become more complex, regimen adherence becomes more important. Parents, caregivers, and providers need to have an understanding of developmentally and cognitively appropriate goals as children begin to perform more self-care skills. Studies reporting age-dependent acquisition of skills imply that cognitive and psychosocial development may mediate self-care skill mastery.[4] Numerous studies have confirmed that early transition of self-care skills and inappropriate expectations from children have led to poor diabetes control. Not only have they led to poor glycemic outcomes but they have also been associated with impeding future skill acquisition.[3] It is important to have a clear understanding of the cognitive and motor skills necessary for children to develop a sense of autonomy with the various tasks associated with diabetes management (**Table 2**).[6]

DIABETES-RELATED SELF-CARE TASKS AND COGNITIVE NEEDS
Self–Blood Glucose Monitoring

Self–blood glucose monitoring is the cornerstone of diabetes management. It helps to evaluate the other components of diabetes management such as medication dosing and the response of the body to physical activity and dietary intake. For a child with diabetes, the physical task of self–blood glucose monitoring requires fine motor skills typically not fully developed before 5 years of age.[4] Cognitive skills related to self–blood glucose monitoring include the ability to understand numeric ordering/serialization and basic mathematical skills to understand and interpret the results. According to Piaget,[7] these cognitive skills are not mastered before elementary school-age years. Although some children may master the technical tasks related to blood glucose monitoring at an early age (4–6 years), many studies have found that relinquishing these tasks too early can lead to inconsistent care and have a negative impact on glucose control.[3]

Insulin/Medication Administration

Insulin administration is necessary for children with type 1 diabetes and often used initially in the management of type 2 diabetes in children. The most common insulin regimen is basal-bolus therapy. It is frequently used because it closely mimics the normal response of the body to CHO intake and energy expenditure. Components of insulin dosing include a basal insulin dose (glargine/detemir) and a bolus dose (lispro/aspart/glulisine), which is calculated from an insulin/CHO ratio and correction factor, used to treat hyperglycemia.

Table 2
Developmental milestones

Age (y)	Behavior Routines	Physical Development	Emotional Development	Cognitive Development	Social Development
3–5	Working toward independence, still needing comfort Spending more time away from home/interacting with environment	Developing and refining motor skills	May display emotional extremes (tantrums) Egocentric	Beginning number and word recognition Learns to count and understand the meaning of numbers	Increasing interactions with children More cooperative play Loosely understands rules
6	Increasingly independent	Developing muscle coordination	Developing skills to handle emotional extremes Has difficulty handling setbacks and losses	Developing basic mathematical skills Beginning to read and write Beginning to understand 'more' or 'less'; 'good', and 'bad' Concrete thought process	Increasing social interactions Improving social skills Beginning to develop friendships
7	Growing more self-sufficient, but needs reminders	Motor skills becoming more precise Increased coordination and balance	More capable of handling surprises and transition Still lack self-control	Inquisitive Asking questions and seeking answers about encounters with people they meet Enjoys mentoring younger children	Friendships important Forming bonds with teachers Beginning to care about opinions of others
8	Daily routines influenced by personality and experiences	Increased muscle coordination and muscle control	Beginning to show more sophisticated and complex emotions and social interactions	Vocabulary and language skills becoming more complex and sophisticated Beginning to express opinions Developing early critical thinking skills	Developing close friendships Enjoys school Values relationships with peers/classmates

Age					
9	Developing early organization skills; Accepts increased responsibilities at home	Stronger, smoother muscle control; May experience beginning puberty	Better at handling frustrations and conflict; Developing strong desire to fit in; Can develop anxiety issues as real fears replace fantasy fears	Beginning to show ability to think critically; Improved mathematical, writing, and verbal skills	Influenced by parent behavior (role model); Strong sense of right and wrong; Becoming more socially conscious; Rudimentary peer pressure may become issue
10–11	Focused and likes to follow schedules; Manages daily responsibilities and activities (except for personal care)	May experience puberty; Risk for body image issues	Able to handle conflict; Able to work in groups; Less egocentric; Focused on school, friends, and extracurricular activities	Beginning abstract thought process; Developing use of logic to problem solve; Developing deductive reasoning skills; More refined organizational strategies	Developing ability to understand multiple viewpoints; Shows empathy toward others
12–18	Capable of managing self-care skills; Risk-taking behaviors emerging; Generally, suboptimal nutrition	Significant growth; Puberty; Increased strength and endurance	Developing autonomy and independence from family; Has sense of immortality and invincibility; Variable emotions	Develops ability to reason abstractly; Problem-solving skills refined; Able to compare and contrast; Developing ability to formulate and consider multiple hypotheses	Vulnerable to peer pressure; Overly romanticized view of world; Spending longer periods in cyberworld

Adapted from Refs.[14–17]

Insulin administration not only requires fine motor manual dexterity to manipulate the various administration devices (syringe/vial, pen device, pump) but also requires the understanding of cause and effect of behaviors related to insulin administration. The manual dexterity needed to manipulate the various insulin administration devices is not often developed before the late school-age years (11–12 years of age).[7,8] Appropriate insulin dosing and administration also require the child to have more advanced mathematical skills including addition/subtraction, multiplication and division, and basic ratio proportion calculation.[7] Insulin doses are determined by calculating an insulin/CHO ratio. They also require the cognitive ability to understand timing of insulin dose related to meal/activity and dose calculations and the ability to determine any necessary dose changes related to dietary intake, activity, and insulin sensitivity. These skills are typically not developed before early adolescence or midadolescence.[3,7]

Many oral agents may cause hypoglycemia if dietary intake or energy expenditure are not taken into consideration when dosing. The child with diabetes requires an understanding of cause and effect and schedule of medication dosing and the ability to determine any dose adjustment related to changes in dietary intake and physical activity. These skills are typically poorly developed before early adolescence.[3]

CHO Counting

CHO counting is the recommended method of meal planning for diabetes management.[9] CHO counting requires modest mathematical skills similar to calculating insulin doses in addition to an understanding of cause and effect, categorization, and measurement skills, which are skills not typically acquired before early adolescence.[7] Basic CHO counting skills such as determining portion size and label reading can be introduced during the late school-age years. Although beginning skills related to CHO counting can be taught during school-age years, the abstract thinking skills necessary to adjust CHO intake for changes in activity and insulin sensitivity are not acquired before midadolescence.[3,7]

Hypoglycemia Detection/Management

Hypoglycemia may occur as a complication of insulin therapy or use of some oral agents. Symptoms occur due to inadequate glucose to the brain, resulting in impaired function. The level of blood glucose low enough to define hypoglycemia is different for different people (young children vs older adolescent), in different circumstances (before exercise or bedtime), and for different purposes (during illness). Before 6 to 7 years of age, children with diabetes have a developmental, hypoglycemic unawareness.[10,11] At this age, they lack the cognitive ability to recognize and respond to hypoglycemia symptoms.[2] They also lack the understanding of appropriate management or treatment of hypoglycemia, because of their concrete thinking process. For example, if a child treats their hypoglycemia until they feel better they may overconsume CHOs during the symptomatic period common with hypoglycemia. Having an understanding of cause and effect as well as the cognitive ability associated with abstract thinking is needed to understand the appropriate management skills necessary to prevent rebound hyperglycemia.[7] As children develop the ability to understand cause and effect during the elementary school-age years, they become more accurate in recognizing activities or events during which they are more likely to develop hypoglycemia.[3] They are also able to understand the basic concepts of treatment strategies. However, the abstract thinking needed to fully understand how to take preventive measures to lessen the risk of hypoglycemia does not fully develop until early adolescence.

Hyperglycemia Detection/Management

Hyperglycemia can cause significant problems in children with diabetes. It can be caused by a mismatch between medication administration and dietary intake, insulin omission, or illness, among other causes. Similar to hypoglycemia symptoms, children younger than 6 to 7 years have difficulty detecting symptoms associated with hyperglycemia. Because of concrete thinking skills associated with the school-age years, the younger child has difficulty understanding the implications of hyperglycemia, including the risk of ketones and dehydration. The abstract thinking process needed to understand the implications of hyperglycemia as well as how to take measures to prevent hyperglycemia is often not well developed until midadolescence.[7]

Emergency Management

For most of the childhood years, children with diabetes require assistance with management of emergent situations such as severe hypoglycemia, illness, and management of ketones. Hypoglycemia often causes transient cognitive impairment. Before midadolescence, many children lack the cognitive ability to anticipate risk and implications of severe hypoglycemia. During periods of illness, cognitive abilities such as cause and effect and early abstract thinking are necessary to understand the implications of illness and impact on diabetes control. These skills are not well developed before early adolescence. Treatment of illnesses and management of insulin and dietary intake all require abstract thinking not fully developed before midadolescence. Similar skills are needed to manage ketones and the risk of deteriorating metabolic control, particularly those on insulin pump therapy.

Exercise

Daily exercise or play is recommended for children with diabetes. Exercise can improve overall glycemic control, yet it also offers an inherent risk of hypoglycemia development as a result of improved insulin use. Cognitive skills necessary to fully understand the relationship of activity, meal timing, and medication administration are not developed until midadolescence. Not until the child has the ability of abstract thinking and an understanding of cause and effect are they able to learn to anticipate hypoglycemia and make necessary changes in medication dosing or CHO consumption to minimize the risk. Before midadolescence, children with diabetes often require assistance in anticipating their metabolic response to changes in activity.

TRANSITION OF RESPONSIBILITIES FOR DIABETES-RELATED SELF-CARE

Most studies assessing the specific age at which children are capable of assuming many of the diabetes-related self-care tasks were conducted in the 1990s.[4,12] Although the age at which children should assume self-care responsibilities for the management of their disease is not clear in many studies, it is important for a child's cognitive development and developmental stage to be taken into account when considering transition of diabetes-related self-care tasks to children and adolescents.[12] It is also important for parental involvement in diabetes care to continue throughout the transition of care. Lack of parent support during the transition of diabetes-related self-care tasks can have devastating effects on metabolic outcomes, consistency in care, and family conflict.[13]

Inappropriate expectations for acquiring self-care skills related to diabetes management by children can have a significant impact on diabetes control and may also impede further acquisition of self-care skills.[4] Entrusting a child to be autonomous in their self-care daily skills before they are developmentally or cognitively capable may interfere with their ability to meet glycemic management goals. Conversely, not allowing a child with the cognitive ability to participate in their personal diabetes care can lead to behaviors of excessive dependence on others to meet management goals. It is important that the management regimen and self-care expectations for the child with diabetes consider the developmental age and cognitive development to ensure the best situation by which to meet glycemic/management goals.

DEVELOPMENTAL STAGES AND TASKS BY AGE-GROUP (PSYCHOSOCIAL/COGNITIVE)

Children are in a continuous state of change in regards to growth and development (**Table 3**). There are various tasks that should be mastered as the child develops.[14–17] Areas of task mastery include development of intellectual abilities and social-emotional development.

Table 3
Cognitive skills and diabetes-related self-care tasks

Self-Care Task	Cognitive Skills Needed for Independence	Typical Age Skill is Acquired
Self–blood glucose monitoring	Fine motor skills Understanding of numeric ordering Numeric place value	May be able to perform fingerstick by 4–5 y of age Ability to interpret results not typical until school-age years
Insulin/medication administration	Fine motor skills/manual dexterity Advanced mathematical skills Understanding of cause and effect Abstract thinking (anticipate dose change)	Self-administration of insulin typically by 10–12 y of age Dose calculations typically by early adolescence Ability to anticipate dose change needs by midadolescence
CHO counting	Mathematical skills Understanding of cause and effect Categorization and measurement skills Abstract thinking (anticipate change)	Categorization and measurement skills emerge during mid school-age years Skills needed to adjust intake needs do not typically emerge before adolescence
Hypoglycemia management	Ability to recognize symptoms Understanding of cause and effect Abstract thinking (anticipate/prevent event)	Symptom recognition not reliable before school-age years Skills needed to adjust intake needs do not typically emerge before adolescence
Hyperglycemia management	Ability to recognize symptoms Understanding of cause and effect Abstract thinking (anticipate/prevent event)	Symptom recognition not reliable before school-age years Skills needed to adjust intake needs do not typically emerge before adolescence
Emergency management	Understanding of cause and effect Abstract thinking (anticipate/manage/prevent event)	Skills needed to anticipate risk and use management strategies not well developed before midadolescence
Exercise	Understanding of cause and effect Abstract thinking (anticipate/manage/prevent event)	Skills needed to evaluate impact of exercise on glycemic control, medications, and dietary intake are not well developed before midadolescence

Data from Refs.[7,14–17]

Toddler/Preschool Years (1 Year–5 Years)

According to Erikson,[6] there are 2 primary psychosocial tasks that toddlers strive to master. First, toddlers work toward separating themselves from the parent/primary caregiver and establishing themselves as an individual by developing a sense of autonomy. Second, they work to acquire a sense of mastery of the environment and their interaction with their environment. When striving for a sense of autonomy, toddlers and preschoolers often test for limitations as they struggle for a sense of control over their environment.[6] In the child with diabetes, these behaviors may manifest themselves as a refusal to cooperate with diabetes-related activities such as glucose monitoring. Conflicts over food such as snacking and food choices may also arise, which may interfere with the parent's ability to meet glycemic goals.

Emotionally, toddlers and preschoolers may show extremes in behaviors, including temper tantrums, as they adjust to contradictions in anticipated responses from their environment. Egocentrism, common in this age-group, also feeds into those extreme behaviors. Parents of young children with diabetes have to learn to differentiate between normal behavior extremes and symptoms of hypoglycemia manifesting itself as behavior change.

Cognitively, toddlers and preschoolers are developing a beginning understanding of measures such as good or bad or more or less. The cognitive thinking process of the toddler and preschooler is concrete. Because of this concrete thought process, the young child with diabetes may perceive that their blood glucose level is representative of their behavior (ie, 'If my blood sugar is "bad", that means I am "bad"'). Caregivers need to be cognizant of their concrete thinking process when evaluating glucose levels to not label the result as good or bad. Toddlers and preschoolers are also beginning to learn to recognize, count, and understand the meaning of numbers as well as developing early skills in reading and writing.[7]

School-Age Years (6–12 Years)

During the school-age years, children strive to develop a sense of industry through the accomplishment of new tasks.[6] School-age children are learning to move from time spent at home to time spent in the school setting, as well as building self-esteem and forging friendships. Through social interactions, they begin to develop a sense of pride in their abilities and accomplishments. School-age children strive to master new skills and emotionally strive to please others.[12] For the child with diabetes, these behaviors may present as the willingness to become independent with their diabetes-related care. It is important for caregivers to be aware that although the children desire to be independent in their diabetes management, they lack the cognitive skills to be successful in their independence. Children who are given too much independence in their care are often unable to appropriately manage their diabetes. Caregivers should allow the child to perform components of their care in which they can be successful. As the school-age child develops cognitive skills that offer them the ability to master simple diabetes-related tasks, they can then be encouraged to slowly assume more responsibility for their care. Caregivers and health professionals need to keep in mind that cognitive ability and not chronologic age should be considered when determining mastery of diabetes-related self-care tasks by the child with diabetes.

The school environment offers an opportunity to assist the school-age child with the building of self-esteem and a sense of accomplishment. Children with diabetes should be encouraged to fully participate in school-related activities and extracurricular activities, as their schedule allows. Participation in extracurricular activities helps to foster the formation of friendships as well as boost self-esteem by offering a sense of accomplishment. Medication administration and dietary strategies should be flexible to account for variability in schedule and degree of physical activity.

Emotionally, school-age children are better at handling changes in schedules and disappointment than their toddler/preschool counterparts. They are beginning to understand their own feelings and consequences of their actions. During the school-age years, children learn to behave according to an appropriate standard of behavior without direct supervision. For the child with diabetes, this developmental characteristic may manifest itself as the desire to please adults or avoid negative consequences from undesired behaviors. During the early school-age years, children may perceive their level of glycemic control as a reflection of their behavior. For example, if they are extensively questioned regarding the cause of an increased blood sugar level, they may be likely to fabricate subsequent glucose values so as to avoid perceived negative consequences.

Cognitively, school-age children are mastering numerous academic skills.[7] They continue to think concretely and in a unidirectional manner. Their thoughts are based on real and concrete experiences. During the school-age years, children begin to engage in classification and serial ordering and become adept at science and mathematics. Children at this age also begin to show conservation.[7] For children with diabetes, the development of conservation skills allows them to understand portion sizes and rudimentary CHO counting skills. Toward the later school-age years, the mastery of serial ordering and the understanding of numeric place value allow the child with diabetes to better understand blood glucose values and early understanding of activity and the impact of dietary intake on glycemic control. Parents, caregivers, and health professionals should encourage developmentally, age-appropriate skills to build self-esteem and independent behaviors.[6] It is important that the school-age child with diabetes be supported in their attainment of self-care skills, yet the responsibility for glycemic management remains with the parent/caregiver.

Adolescence (13–19 Years)

Adolescence is a time of significant transition physically, emotionally, and cognitively. Significant changes in growth and physical development occur during adolescence, which can affect dietary strategies and medication needs of adolescents with diabetes. Adolescents strive to meet 2 primary psychosocial goals. Establishing an identity is probably the most important task associated with adolescence.[6] They begin to integrate the opinions of others (caregivers, parents, and friends) with their own beliefs. They strive to blend with their peer group and are self-conscious of how others perceive their behaviors. For adolescents with diabetes, this desire to integrate with their peer group and self-conscious thoughts may result in mismanagement of diabetes-related tasks (delayed/omitted glucose monitoring, insulin dosing delay/omission, or poor dietary food choices). Offering flexibility in monitoring, dietary regimens, and medication dosing may alleviate these issues and assist the adolescent in fitting their diabetes management tasks into their schedule/peer group activities.

The attainment of autonomy as shown through becoming independent in their thoughts and actions is another primary task associated with adolescence.[6] Through their cognitive advances and ability, adolescents with diabetes become more capable of taking an active role in their diabetes management. It is important that caregivers and health care providers recognize the fine line between the psychosocial and cognitive ability to assume more independent self-care behaviors and the noncompliance that can develop if too much independence is thrust on the adolescent.

Emotionally, adolescents have a heightened sense of self-consciousness.[18] They tend to believe that everyone is as concerned about their thoughts and feelings and often feel as if everyone is looking at them. Adolescents also tend to believe that no one has ever experienced similar situations or feelings. Feelings of invincibility also emerge during adolescence. For the adolescent with diabetes, these emotional behaviors may lead to risk-taking behaviors with regards to their diabetes management (insulin omission, noncompliance with monitoring and dietary strategies) in addition to normal adolescent risk-taking behaviors. They may have dramatic descriptions of how they feel about their diabetes and may become resistant to diabetes-related self-care tasks.

Cognitively, adolescents are developing abstract thought process and advanced reasoning skills.[7] The development of abstract thinking and advanced reasoning skills allows adolescents to logically consider multiple options and possibilities when considering their actions or behaviors. Adolescents are developing proficiency in evaluating hypothetical situations as well. For the adolescent with diabetes, these more complex cognitive skills allow for the capability of assuming more responsibility for many of their diabetes-related self-care. Having more sophisticated reasoning skills permits the adolescent with diabetes to manage more complex regimens and thus to plan and account for variability in their daily schedule.

INTERVENTIONS TO MINIMIZE ISSUES AND ASSIST WITH APPROPRIATE TRANSITION OF DIABETES-RELATED SKILLS

Numerous steps can be taken to minimize difficulties often encountered during transition of diabetes-related self-care tasks from parent to child (**Table 4**). Integration of normal developmental tasks and cognitive skill development with self-care skill expectations lessens struggles between the child with diabetes and their caregivers.

Toddlers and preschoolers are striving for autonomy and self-confidence.[6] They fear loss of control over a situation. This fear may manifest itself as refusal to cooperate with diabetes-related self-care tasks. To alleviate these behaviors, positive reinforcement should be offered when the child cooperates with the diabetes regimen. The child should be offered choices when possible to give them a sense of control. Diabetes care should be kept routine around meals, snacks, and activities. The child should be allowed to assist with self-care activities, if they desire (such as a fingerstick when monitoring blood glucose levels). All diabetes-related care is to be provided by the caregiver. The toddler and preschooler should not be personally responsible for any self-care activities.

The school-age child begins to understand cause and effect in addition to the development of numerous cognitive, athletic, and social skills. They are beginning to forge new friend relationships, refine motor skills, and attain new academic skills such as conservation, understanding measurement, numeric place value, and basic mathematical skills.[6,7] School-age children continue to fear a loss of control. However, more frequently, they have a fear of failure or fear of not living up to others' expectations. To alleviate some of these issues, ways can be found to make diabetes regimens flexible to allow for participation in school events and peer activities. Again, choices can be offered when possible and more personal involvement in their diabetes care can be allowed for. Although the adolescents are beginning to develop skills to self-manage their diabetes care, school-age children should always have supervision when performing these skills to ensure safety and management success (**Table 5**).[19]

Table 4
Ways to minimize problems with transition of self-management skills

Age-Group Tasks	Emerging Issues	Suggested Interventions

Toddler/Preschool
  Independence
  Mastery of environment
	Limit testing
	Needing sense of control
	Refusal to cooperate
	Conflict over food
		Support normal
		  developmental tasks
		Allow choices when possible
		  (eg, which injection site,
		  which finger for glucose
		  monitoring)
		Allow to assist with tasks as
		  interested (eg, gathering
		  monitoring supplies,
		  selecting snacks)
		Work around food
		  preferences

School-age
  Separation from parents
  Skill development
  Develop friend
    relationships
  Compare self with others
  School transition
  Reliance on others outside
    family
	School transition
	Social events
	Emerging self-esteem
	Influence of peer reaction
	Emerging responsibility for
	  care
		Ensure a written plan for
		  school identifying roles for
		  self-care management
		Allow full participation in
		  age-appropriate activities
		Increase involvement in care
		Encourage self-advocacy
		Share disease information
		  with peer group
		Encourage flexibility in
		  regimens to support
		  activities

Adolescence
  Separation from family
  Independence
  Identity development
  Limit testing
  Impulse control
  Friends primary support
  Increase responsibility for
    care
	Parent conflict
	Limit testing
	Peer influence on behaviors
	Substance use here-and-now
	  attitude
	Poor or inconsistent eating/
	  sleep patterns
	Poor self-management
		Allow increased control by
		  adolescent, yet continued
		  involvement by caregiver/
		  parent
		Build support among family
		  and friends
		Train friends about health
		  care routine
		Build self-efficacy and positive
		  health beliefs
		Set clear expectations and use
		  behavior contracts
		Communicate, communicate,
		  communicate

Adapted from Erikson EH. Childhood and society. 2nd edition. New York: W.W. Norton and Company; 1993; and Piaget J, Inhelder B. The psychology of the child. 2nd edition. New York: Basic Books; 1969. p. 255–61.

Adolescents are becoming more abstract and logical in their thinking.[7] They are striving for a sense of self-identity and have feelings of indestructibility, yet they fear being different from their peers and the loss of control over various situations.[6] Because these psychosocial tasks and fears may interfere with an adolescent's ability to independently manage their diabetes, it is important to have continued involvement in care by the parent/caregiver. Consideration can be given to involving a friend in assisting with diabetes management.[19] Negotiating various roles for diabetes management may allow for a sense of control by the adolescent, yet maintain parent/caregiver involvement to ensure that appropriate management skills are being

Table 5
Skills the school-age child may perform

Diabetes Tasks School-Age Child Can Do	Diabetes Tasks School-Age Child Should Not Do
Help check own blood sugar	Be responsible for always understanding when to check blood sugar
Help count CHOs	Be left to count CHOs independently at all times
When ready, give own injection	Give injection without supervision
Write down in record book	Be responsible for keeping all records
Tell you (adult) when they feel low	Always know how to anticipate or prevent a low
Start to learn what their insulin doses are	Know when and how to make dose changes
Do the maths with you when calculating a dose	Always be expected to calculate insulin doses
Check ketones, with help from caregiver	Be left alone, or know what to do when sick

From Children's Hospitals and Clinics of Minnesota. Age-appropriate diabetes care [online]. 2009. Available at: http://www.childrensmn.org/web/diabetes/200928.pdf. Accessed August 30, 2012; with permission.

adequately performed to ensure glycemic control. The adolescent can be encouraged to take responsibility for independence in other areas of life; however, the diabetes management should be protected from similar expectations.[19]

SUMMARY

The goal of managing diabetes in childhood is to assist the child in becoming a physically healthy and emotionally mature adult, free from complications associated with diabetes.[3] Gradual achievement of self-care independence occurs as developmental changes evolve during childhood. It is important to be cognizant of the cognitive, psychosocial, and emotional skills needed to assist the child with diabetes in achieving age-appropriate self-care independence. By having an understanding of normal growth and development as it relates to diabetes self-care tasks, appropriate expectations for the child with diabetes can be determined. Appropriate expectations and support in the acquisition of self-management skills can help the child with diabetes move to self-care independence.

REFERENCES

1. Centers for Disease Control and Prevention. Children and diabetes search for diabetes in youth [on-line]. 2011. Available at: http://www.cdc.gov/diabetes/projects/diab_children.htm. Accessed July 20, 2012.
2. US Department of Health and Human Services' National Diabetes Education Program. Overview of diabetes in children and adolescence [on-line]. 2011. Available at: http://ndep.nih.gov/media/youth_factsheet.pdf. Accessed August 5, 2012.
3. Clarke WL. Behavioral challenges in the management of childhood diabetes. J Diabetes Sci Technol 2011;5(2):225–8.
4. Wysocki T, Meinhold PA, Abrams KC, et al. Parental and professional estimates of self-care independence of children and adolescents with IDDM. Diabetes Care 1992;15(1):43–52.
5. American Diabetes Association. Standards of medical care in diabetes–2012 position statement. Diabetes Care 2012;35(Suppl 1):S11–63.

6. Erikson EH. Childhood and society. 2nd edition. New York: WW Norton; 1993.

7. Piaget J, Inhelder B. The psychology of the child. 2nd edition. New York: Basic Books; 1969.

8. Naughten E, Smith MA, Baum JD. At what age do diabetic children give their own injections? Am J Dis Child 1982;136(8):690–2.

9. Husney A. Diabetes in children: Counting carbs [on-line]. 2010. Available at: http://diabetes.webmd.com/carbohydrate-counting-for-children-with-diabetes#. Accessed August 4, 2012.

10. Clarke W, Jones T, Rewers A, et al. Assessment and management of hypoglycemia in children and adolescents with diabetes. Pediatr Diabetes 2009; 10(Suppl 12):134–45.

11. National Institutes of Health's National Institutes of Diabetes, Digestive and Kidney Diseases. National diabetes information clearinghouse: Hypoglycemia [on-line]. 2008. Available at: http://diabetes.niddk.nih.gov/dm/pubs/hypoglycemia/. Accessed August 5, 2012.

12. Anderson BJ, Laffel LM. Behavioral and psychosocial research with school-aged children with type 1 diabetes. Diabetes Spectr 1997;10:4.

13. Anderson BJ. Family conflict and diabetes management in youth: clinical lessons from child development and diabetes research. Diabetes Spectr 2004;17(1): 22–6.

14. National Center on Birth Defects and Developmental Disabilities. Preschoolers: child development (3-5 years old) [on-line]. 2009. Available at: http://www. medicinenet.com/preschoolers_child_development/article.htm. Accessed August 13, 2012.

15. Mersch J. Young children: child development (6-8 years old) [on-line]. 2009. Available at: http://www.medicinenet.com/young_children_child_development/article. htm. Accessed August 13, 2012.

16. Mersch J. Tween: child development (9-11 years old) [on-line]. 2009. Available at: http://www.medicinenet.com/tween_child_development/article.htm. Accessed August 7, 2012.

17. Mersch J. Teen: child development (12-17 years old) [on-line]. 2009. Available at: http://www.medicinenet.com/teen_child_development/article.htm. Accessed August 7, 2012.

18. Huebner A. Adolescent growth and development [on-line]. 2009. Available at: http://pubs.ext.vt.edu/350/350-850/350-850.html. Accessed August 23, 2012.

19. Children's Hospitals and Clinics of Minnesota. Age-appropriate diabetes care [on-line]. 2009. Available at: http://www.childrensmn.org/web/diabetes/200928. pdf. Accessed August 30, 2012.

Implementation of a Clinical Practice Guideline for Identification of Microalbuminuria in the Pediatric Patient with Type 1 Diabetes

Kathleen A. Montgomery, MSN, CRNP[a],*, Sarah J. Ratcliffe, PhD[b],
H. Jorge Baluarte, MD[c], Kathryn M. Murphy, PhD, RN[d],
Steven Willi, MD[e], Terri H. Lipman, PhD, CRNP, FAAN[f]

KEYWORDS

- Clinical practice guidelines • Children • Diabetic nephropathy

KEY POINTS

- Screening for microalbuminuria (MA) in the pediatric population is important because of the significant physiologic, psychosocial, and financial costs of end-stage renal disease in people with type 1 diabetes.
- This article emphasizes the need to screen all children with type 1 diabetes annually beginning at the 1-year anniversary of diagnosis.
- When discussing laboratory results and the need for repeat testing, the clinician should provide education about the importance of continuing the screening process.
- Because black children are more likely to have persistent MA, attention must be paid to assuring that this population is referred for screening, and, if needed, that follow-up testing has been completed.
- This study underscores the importance of developing clinical practice guidelines (CPGs) to guide nurses in evidence-based practice.
- The ultimate goal of using CPGs in children with chronic medical conditions is to assist the provider in identifying children at risk for complications, encouraging optimal disease management, and assuring appropriate referral to a specialist if necessary.

[a] Division of Endocrinology and Diabetes, The Children's Hospital of Philadelphia, 34th and Civic Center Boulevard, Philadelphia, PA 19104, USA; [b] Department of Biostatistics and Epidemiology, Perelman School of Medicine, University of Pennsylvania, 610 Blockley Hall, 423 Guardian Drive, Philadelphia, PA 19104-6021, USA; [c] Division of Nephrology, The Children's Hospital of Philadelphia, Perelman School of Medicine, University of Pennsylvania, 34th and Civic Center Boulevard, Philadelphia, PA 19104, USA; [d] Division of Endocrinology and Diabetes, The Children's Hospital of Philadelphia, University of Pennsylvania School of Nursing, 34th and Civic Center Boulevard, Philadelphia, PA 19104, USA; [e] Division of Endocrinology and Diabetes, The Children's Hospital of Philadelphia, Perelman School of Medicine, University of Pennsylvania, 34th and Civic Center Boulevard, Philadelphia, PA 19104, USA; [f] Division of Endocrinology and Diabetes, The Children's Hospital of Philadelphia, University of Pennsylvania School of Nursing, 418 Curie Boulevard, Philadelphia, PA 19104, USA
* Corresponding author.
E-mail address: montgomery@email.chop.edu

Nurs Clin N Am 48 (2013) 343–352
http://dx.doi.org/10.1016/j.cnur.2013.01.003
0029-6465/13/$ – see front matter © 2013 Elsevier Inc. All rights reserved.

INTRODUCTION

Developing an evidence-based practice culture can be challenging in a large organization with complex systems and multiple team members providing care. There are several obstacles to overcome before a successful evidence-based practice approach can be initiated. Inherent in an evidence-based approach is the collection and analysis of data related to practice guidelines and the development of interventions to improve patient care based on empirical and clinical data.

Clinical practice guidelines (CPG) are evidence based, and are designed to provide a structure for the health care provider and patient's family regarding specific clinical circumstances.[1] According to Sackett and colleagues,[2] evidence-based practice is the integrating of "individual clinical expertise with the best available external clinical evidence from systematic research" (p. 71). Evidence-based CPGs strive to improve the quality, outcomes, and cost-effectiveness of health care.[3] The development of CPGs is critical to direct the assessment and management of children with diabetes.

BACKGROUND

Type 1 diabetes mellitus is an autoimmune disease affecting the islet cells of the pancreas, which lose the ability to produce insulin, a hormone needed for normal glucose metabolism. Persons with type 1 diabetes require lifelong administration of insulin by injection or via continuous subcutaneous insulin infusion.[4] Diabetes is one of the most common chronic diseases in school-aged children, affecting about 215,000 people less than 20 years of age in the United States in 2010[4]; it can result in multiple complications and comorbidities that can lead to significant morbidity and mortality. According to the National Diabetes Information Clearinghouse,[4] diabetes is the seventh leading cause of death in the United States and is likely underreported. Long-term complications can include blindness, kidney damage, cardiovascular disease, and neuropathy. A significant aspect of care for persons with diabetes is focused on early detection and prevention of complications through routine screening, adequate blood glucose control, and control of blood pressure and lipid levels. In our diabetes center, screening for diabetes complications and comorbidities was sporadic and varied according to provider preference. In the past several years, the center has been developing and implementing CPGs to assist providers in their attempts to identify incipient diabetes complications.

Screening for diabetic nephropathy was one of the first CPGs developed. Nephropathy is one of the most serious long-term complications of diabetes, and often leads to chronic renal failure, which results in the need for dialysis or kidney transplant. Diabetes is currently the leading single cause of end-stage renal disease in the United States and Europe.[5] Despite significant improvements in care, recent estimates place the prevalence of nephropathy at between 10% and 20% of diabetes patients overall.[6]

The earliest clinical evidence of nephropathy is microalbuminuria (MA), which is the presence of small quantities of albumin in the urine (30–300 mg/24 hours).[5] Albumin is the most common protein found in the urine.[7] Approximately one-third of patients newly diagnosed with type 1 diabetes develop persistent MA within the first 20 years of diabetes.[8] Because prompt treatment of MA may reverse symptoms and delay or prevent complications, it is imperative to detect MA early in patients with diabetes.[9] MA may occur even in young children and in those with diabetes of brief duration.[10] The American Diabetes Association (ADA) and National Kidney Foundation recommend screening for MA in children and adolescents using a spot urine sample for microalbumin/creatinine ratio (MACR).[11] A first morning sample is recommended, but a random sample is considered acceptable.

Several factors present challenges for developing a CPGs for MA screening in children with diabetes, most notably false-positive results. In a normal pediatric population, as many as 10% of school-aged children test positive for proteinuria by urinary dipstick, but only 0.1% are positive when retested.[12] Between 30% and 50% of children with proteinuria may have transient proteinuria, and, of those with persistent proteinuria, most have a benign condition called orthostatic proteinuria.[13] In addition, measurement of MACR may be affected by exercise, illness, hypertension, marked hyperglycemia, and diurnal patterns.[14] Thus, some children with diabetes have false-positive screening results.

PURPOSE

This study evaluated provider adherence to a CPG in identifying children with MA, whether a random spot urine specimen was effective in the identification of MA, and the demographic factors associated with persistent MA. This article presents an overview of the infrastructure and processes that are paramount to providing evidence-based care in a large urban pediatric center.

SAMPLE AND METHODS

The Diabetes Center for Children at The Children's Hospital of Philadelphia follows 2100 children with type 1 diabetes and comprises 20 nurse practitioners and 13 physicians who practice in 6 sites in the Philadelphia area. During the 1-year period of the study, 1566 children and adolescents with type 1 diabetes were evaluated in the Diabetes Center.

PROCEDURES
Development of a CPG

To formulate a CPG for the assessment of MA in children with type 1 diabetes, an interest group was formed, consisting of 2 diabetes nurse practitioners and an attending physician in endocrinology. Existing clinical guidelines from the ADA and the National Kidney Foundation for the assessment of MA in adult patients with diabetes were reviewed. In addition, literature was reviewed using the search terms type 1 diabetes, microalbuminuria, diabetic nephropathy, and pediatrics. In addition, benchmarking was done, contacting the 5 largest pediatric diabetes centers in the country to discuss their method of screening for MA in children with diabetes. Once the data from these 3 sources were compiled, a pediatric nephrologist was added to the MA interest group. Through a series of meetings, a draft CPG was developed. The guideline, along with a review of the literature on MA in children with diabetes, was presented to 20 diabetes nurse practitioners and 5 diabetes physicians. Feedback was provided from the diabetes team and the guidelines were revised. The final CPG was placed on the hospital's diabetes intranet site for ready access at all practice locations.

Description of the CPG

Recommendations of the CPG included screening for MA with an MACR test using a random urine sample at the 1-year anniversary of diagnosis. For ease of collection, the CPG suggested screening with a random urine specimen obtained at the time of a diabetes outpatient visit. For those who screened positive for MA, the CPG recommended that the result be confirmed with a repeat MACR using a first morning sample within 3 to 6 months of the original screen. Those children who continued to screen positive on follow-up testing were to be referred to a nephrologist for further evaluation.

Diabetes Center Database Review

After the CPG had been used for 1 year, a retrospective review of the Diabetes Center database of all children evaluated in a 1-year period was performed. Data were collected on all children with type 1 diabetes who had a documented MA screening during the study period. Data were collected on the subjects' age, sex, race, and duration of diabetes.

Evaluation of Provider Adherence to the CPG

For those children with a positive random screen, the database was reviewed to determine whether a first morning urine was ordered within 3 to 6 months. The database was also reviewed to determine documentation of a follow-up plan, results of subsequent tests, and the final disposition of the patient (eg, return to routine screening, referral to a nephrologist).

Evaluation of Random Spot Urine to Predict MA

Data were analyzed to determine the positive predictive value of an MA screen, using random spot urine in identifying children with MA, confirmed by a first morning void.

Statistical Analysis

Descriptive statistics were calculated for all children with a positive screening test and by whether they had a positive confirmatory test (persistent MA) or not. The persistent and nonpersistent groups were compared using the Student t-test or Fisher exact test, as appropriate. The positive predictive value of the screening test was calculated. All analyses were performed in Stata MP 10.1.

RESULTS
Adherence to the CPG

Of the 1566 children who were evaluated in the Diabetes Center during the study period, 776 (49.5%) patients were screened for MA. A total of 65 children screened positive and required a follow-up urine test. A first morning void for MACR was ordered by the provider on 54 (83%) of the children who screened positive, and a follow-up test result value was documented on 17 (26%) children, within 6 months of the original screening test, as recommended by the guideline. However, a follow-up result was documented on 57 (88%) children within 12 months of the initial positive result.

Prevalence and Predictive Value of a Positive Screen

Of the 776 children evaluated for the presence of MA with a random spot urine specimen for MACR, a normal MACR was noted in 711 (91.6%). Sixty-five children (8.4%) had an increased random spot MACR: 19 boys and 46 girls. Patients with a positive screen ranged in age from 3.9 to 21 years, with a mean age of 13.3 years. Forty-two children were white, 14 were black, and 9 were of other/unknown races. Duration of diabetes ranged from 3 months to 17 years. Sixteen children less than 11 years of age had initial positive screening results for MA.

Of the 65 children with increased spot MACR, 41 (63%) were normal on repeat testing, whereas 16 remained increased, showing that a random spot urine had a positive predictive value of 27.6%. Eight children had no follow-up result documented (**Fig. 1**).

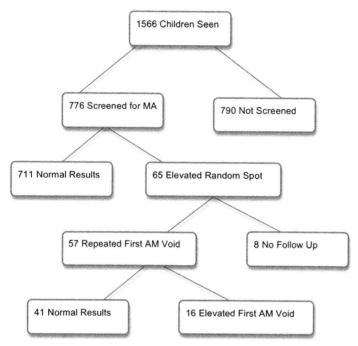

Fig. 1. Adherence to CPGs: screening for MA.

Children with Persistently Increased MACR

There were 2 boys and 14 girls with persistently increased MACR. Eight were white, 7 were African American, and 1 was of another race. Ages ranged from 7.3 to 18.7 years (mean 13.3 years), and the duration of diabetes ranged from 0.9 to 17 years (mean 5.4 years). Black children were significantly more likely to have persistently increased MACR ($P<.05$) (**Table 1**). There were 9 children (56%) who had persistently increased MA, but who had duration of diabetes of less than 5 years.

Table 1				
Disparities in persistent MA by race and sex				
		Persistent MA		
	All (n = 53)[a]	**Yes (n = 15)**	**No (n = 38)**	**P value**
Age (y)	12.7 ± 3.3	13.2 ± 3.0	12.5 ± 3.5	.511
Race				.046
White	39 (73.6)	8 (53.3)	31 (81.6)	
Black	14 (26.4)	7 (46.7)	7 (18.4)	
Female	39 (73.6)	13 (86.7)	26 (68.4)	.188
Duration of diabetes (y)	4.8 ± 3.3	5.4 ± 4.7	4.5 ± 2.5	.501

There is a significant association between race and children who are persistent for MA. Black children have almost 4-fold higher odds of having persistent MA compared with white children (odds ratio = 3.88, 95% confidence interval= 1.05–14.28).

[a] Nine children who were of other/unknown races were excluded from this analysis.

DISCUSSION
Adherence to the CPG

Only half of the children eligible to be screened for MA were screened during the study period. It is unclear to what extent this deficit is attributable to patient, provider, or system issues, all of which might have presented barriers to CPG implementation. Some screening tests ordered in the calendar year of the study may not have appeared in our database until the following year and therefore were not captured in our data. Collins and colleagues[15] outline several reasons why attempts to change practice can fail, including:

> "...When the individual or group perceive the change as a threat...; don't understand why the practice should be changed; receive inadequate education about the change; were not involved in the decisions about the change; believe that the change was not for the better; believe that the potential benefits are not work the effort; believe that the change adversely impacts work flow; and/or believe that too many changes are happening too close and with little planning" (The Evolving Model, paragraph 6).

Of those children who screened positive for MA and required a follow-up first morning urine test, there were fewer MACR results available than were ordered by providers, which indicates that the burden on the patient may be a factor that further impedes guideline adherence. Obtaining a follow-up first morning urine specimen is inconvenient for the patient. Urine must be obtained early in the morning and then stored or promptly brought to a laboratory in an acceptable specimen container. Because of insurance restrictions, many patients have laboratory studies completed at outside commercial laboratories, which delays the reporting of results and data entry. Waitzfelder and colleagues[16] cite cost barriers and inconvenience as factors that may contribute to suboptimal clinical care in youth with diabetes. These factors support our recommendation to initiate screening with a random spot urine specimen at the time of the outpatient visit whenever possible. In light of the barriers to obtaining repeat urine specimens, we extended the data review period to 12 months beyond the initial positive result, and the likelihood of follow-up studies greatly improved.

Over the past 2 decades, a significant body of literature regarding provider adherence to CPGs has emerged.[14,17–19] According to Hysong and colleagues,[19] facilities with a record of successful guideline adherence tend to deliver more timely, individualized, and nonpunitive feedback to providers about their individual guideline adherence, from a perspective of process improvement and professional development rather than one of accountability and punishment for failure.

In our facility, nurse practitioners act as evidence-based practice mentors and are the driving force behind the development and revision of screening guidelines. A part of the nurse practitioner's role as mentor is to provide regular individual feedback to each provider regarding adherence to the CPG. This feedback occurs through the sharing of quarterly reports generated from the diabetes database. Also, regular work group meeting time was incorporated into the Diabetes Center meeting schedule to support all clinicians in this work. The CPGs were reviewed annually at a Diabetes Center group meeting, and there were opportunities for feedback from users to CPG mentors. Users had the opportunity to discuss logistics and limitations of the guideline. In the case of MA screening, several care providers identified that the need for a follow-up study in cases of abnormal initial screens, and the time delay and inconvenience to families, were specific barriers to adherence to the guideline within the designated time frame of 3 to 6 months. Therefore, the CPG was revised to recommend that confirmatory specimens should be available within 3 to 12 months. Additional suggestions to remove the CPG barriers and considerations for implementation are shown in **Table 2**.

Prevalence of a Positive Screen: Evaluation of a Random Spot Urine Specimen as a Valid Screening Test for MA in Children with Type1 Diabetes Mellitus

In our population, most children with type 1 diabetes screened for MA using a random spot urine specimen had normal test results. These data are similar to those reported from the United Kingdom and Ireland showing that 90% of their population of children and adolescents aged 10 to 20 years had normal urine screens using early morning urine samples.[20] A large study of children, adolescents, and adults with type 1 diabetes in Germany and Austria reported normal urine screening tests in 95.6% of patients and persistent abnormal urine tests in 4.3% of patients.[21] Although measurement of MACR using a first morning or random urine sample may differ because of exercise, stress, diurnal variation, and other factors,[22,23] several studies have shown that random urine samples are an accurate estimate of quantitative protein excretion in children[24–26] and adults.[22,23]

Although the positive predictive value of screening with a random urine specimen was low, this type of screening required no additional studies or tracking for the 91.6% of our population who screened negative. For those who screened positive, 28% were correctly identified as needing referral to a nephrologist. Only 5% of the 776 children screened were required to obtain an unnecessary follow-up first AM test.

Guidelines from the ADA and National Kidney Foundation do not recommend screening for MA in children with type 1 diabetes until the child is 10 years of age and/or has had diabetes for 5 years.[11,27] Our data showed that young children and those who have had diabetes for a short duration were still at risk for MA. Other researchers have noted persistent MA in young children with short disease duration.[14,28] If these groups of children were not screened, MA could not have been identified.

Table 2
Suggestions from providers to improve CPG adherence

Suggestion	Whether Implemented	Considerations
Perform urine dipstick at time of visit	No	Questionable sensitivity of urine dipstick in identifying MA
Have patient bring first morning urine sample to each visit	Under consideration (if insurance allows tests to be performed at visit)	Inconvenience of carrying urine throughout the day Patient's insurance may be capitated to a laboratory other than a clinic
Repeat another random spot urine MACR at time of next visit (3 mo)	Yes	Continued issue of possible false-positive results of random spot tests
Mail specimen cup, patient education materials, form letter, and laboratory requisition to patient/parent	Yes	May require ongoing surveillance to ensure patient/family follow-through

There were racial disparities in the prevalence of MA in our population. Black children were almost 4 times more likely to have persistent MA compared with white children, which is similar to the data reported by others.[29] This finding is in line with the disproportionate burden of chronic kidney disease observed in this population.[30] Women were more likely to have persistent MA. Data presented by Holl and colleagues[14] also concluded that female sex was independently related to urinary albumin excretion rate. Raile and colleagues[21] concluded that, in adolescents, female sex increased the risk of MA, whereas, in adults, men were at higher risk of developing MA and overt nephropathy. Moayeri and Dalili[31] concluded that the development of MA is accelerated in girls.

SUMMARY/CLINICAL IMPLICATIONS

Screening for MA in the pediatric population is important because of the significant physiologic, psychosocial, and financial costs of end-stage renal disease in people with type 1 diabetes. Early treatment of MA is inexpensive, and can often slow or even reverse the presence of protein in the urine, thereby preserving kidney function.[32]

Screening with a random spot urine specimen was useful in our population. Collection of random spot urine samples allows the point of care collection of specimens, thereby optimizing the number of children screened and enhancing the convenience to patient, family, and provider. Nonetheless, follow-up is essential in light of the high false-positive rate anticipated with this approach. When discussing laboratory results and the need for repeat testing, the clinician should provide education about the importance of continuing the screening process. To assist clinicians with this endeavor, we created hyperlinks to patient education materials and standardized form letters detailing the parameters for repeat testing within our CPG. In addition, proper specimen cups and laboratory requisition forms were mailed to the patient rather than waiting until the next office visit. To reduce the number of false-positive results, we educated providers on the importance of asking the patient about recent exercise, acute illness, menstruation, and even stressful life events before ordering random spot urine tests. Consideration should be given to delaying the test under these circumstances.

We emphasize the need to screen all children with type 1 diabetes annually, beginning at the 1-year anniversary of diagnosis. Although it is rare to see persistent MA before puberty and with short disease duration,[31] and although it is possible for young children to have MA that is not caused by diabetic nephropathy, it is still critical to identify and refer these children for appropriate evaluation and treatment. Because black children are more likely to have persistent MA, attention must be paid to assuring that this population is referred for screening, and, if needed, that follow-up testing has been completed.

Further education of clinical and data entry staff, revisions to our outpatient clinic records, and ongoing process and outcomes monitoring is needed to support this effort. Regular updates at Diabetes Center meetings, instruction for data entry personnel, and the furnishing of regular provider report cards indicating adherence to the CPG are currently ongoing. Additional review of charts to track results on the children with no documented follow-up is needed. In addition, assessing the contribution of our form revisions to authenticating compliance will be essential as we move toward an electronic medical record.

This study underscores the importance of developing CPGs to guide nurses in evidence-based practice. Use of a CPG for MA screening, management, and evaluation is critical to standardization of care. The ultimate goal of using CPG in children with chronic medical conditions is to assist the provider in identifying children at risk for complications, encouraging optimal disease management, and ensuring appropriate referral to a specialist, if necessary.

REFERENCES

1. Cabana MD, Rand CS, Powe NR, et al. Why don't physicians follow clinical practice guidelines? A framework for improvement. JAMA 1999;282(15):1458–65.
2. Sackett DL, Rosenberg WM, Muir Gray JA, et al. Evidence based medicine: what it is and what it isn't. BMJ 1996;312:71–2.
3. Kenefick H, Lee J, Fleishman V. Improving physician adherence to clinical practice guidelines: barriers and strategies for change. Cambridge (MA): New England Healthcare Institute; 2008.
4. National Diabetes Information Clearinghouse, NIH Publication No 11-3892. Available at: http://diabetes.niddk.nih.gov/dm/pubs/statistics/. Accessed September 12, 2012.
5. American Diabetes Association. Nephropathy in diabetes. Diabetes Care 2004; 27:S79–83. Available at: http://care.diabetsjournals.org/cgi/content/full/diacare; 27/supl_l/s79. Accessed March 2, 2006.
6. Monti MC, Lonsdale JT, Montomoli C, et al. Familial risk factors for microvascular complications and differential male-female risk in a large cohort of American families with type 1 diabetes. J Clin Endocrinol Metab 2007;92(12):4650–5. Available at: jcem.endojournals.org. Accessed January 8, 2008.
7. The Free Dictionary by Farlex. Available at: http://medical-dictionary. thefreedictionary.com/albuminuria. Accessed October 23, 2012.
8. Hovind P, Tarnow L, Rossing P, et al. Predictors for the development of microalbuminuria and macroalbuminuria in patients with type 1 diabetes: inception cohort study. BMJ 2004. Available at: BMJ.com. http://dx.doi.org/10.1136/bmj.38070.450891.FE. Accessed December 8, 2006.
9. Eppens MC, Craig ME, Cusumano J, et al. Prevalence of diabetes complications in adolescents with type 2 compared with type1 diabetes. Diabetes Care 2006; 29:6.
10. Stone ML, Craig ME, Chan AK, et al. Natural history and risk factors for microalbuminuria in adolescents with type 1 diabetes. Diabetes Care 2006;29(9):2072–7.
11. American Diabetes Association. Executive summary: standards of medical care in diabetes 2012. Diabetes Care 2012;35(1):S4–10.
12. Leung AK, Wong AH. Proteinuria in children. Am Fam Physician 2010;82(6): 645–51.
13. Lohgman-Adham M. Evaluating proteinuria in children. Am Fam Physician 1998; 58(5). Available at: http://www.aafp.org/afp/981001ap/loghman.html. Accessed January 19, 2007.
14. Holl RW, Grabert M, Thon A, et al. Urinary excretion of albumin in adolescents with type 1 diabetes. Diabetes Care 1999;22(9):1555–60.
15. Collins PM, Golembeski SM, Selgas M, et al. Clinical excellence through evidence-based practice – a model to guide practice changes. Topics in Advanced Practice Nursing eJournal 2007;7(4). Posted 01/25/2008. Available at: http://www.medscape.com/viewarticle/567682.
16. Waitzfelder B, Pihoker C, Klingensmith G, et al. Adherence to guidelines for youths with diabetes mellitus. Pediatrics 2011;128(3):531–8.
17. Goetz LL, Nelson AL, Guihan M, et al. Provider adherence to implementation of clinical practice guidelines for neurogenic bowel in adults with spinal cord injury. J Spinal Cord Med 2005;28:394–406.

18. Cook D, Giacomini M. The trials and tribulations of clinical practice guidelines. JAMA 1999;281:1950–1.
19. Hysong SJ, Best RG, Pugh JA. Audit and feedback and clinical practice guideline adherence: Making feedback actionable. Implement Sci 2006;1:9. Available at: http://www.implementationscience.com/content/1/1/9. Accessed September 3, 2008.
20. Moore TH, Shield JP. Prevalence of abnormal urinary albumin excretion in adolescents and children with insulin dependent diabetes: the MIDAC study. Arch Dis Child 2000;83:239–43.
21. Raile K, Galler A, Hofer S, et al. Diabetic nephropathy in 27,805 children, adolescents and adults with type 1 diabetes: effect of diabetes duration, A1C, hypertension, dyslipidemia, diabetes onset, and sex. Diabetes Care 2007;30(10):2523–8.
22. Babazono T, Takahashi C, Iwamoto Y. Definition of microalbuminuria in first-morning and random spot urine in diabetic patients. Diabetes Care 2004;27: 1838–9.
23. Khan A, Ahmad TM, Qureshi H, et al. Assessment of proteinuria by using protein: creatinine index in random urine sample. J Pakistan Med Assoc. Available at: http://www.jpma.org.pk/full_article_text.php?article_id=891. Accessed October 23, 2012.
24. Tsai WS, Tsau YK, Chen CH, et al. Correlation between total urinary protein quantitation and random urine sample protein/creatinine ratio in children. J Formos Med Assoc 1991;90(8):760–3.
25. Chang JB, Chen YH, Chu NF. Relationship between single voided urine protein/creatinine ratio and 24-hour urine protein excretion rate among children and adolescents in Taiwan. Zhonghua Yi Xue Za Zhi 2000;63(11):828–32.
26. Assadi FK. Quantitation of microalbuminuria using random urine samples. Pediatr Nephrol 2002;17:107–10.
27. Silverstein J, Klingensmith G, Copeland K, et al. Care of children and adolescents with type 1 diabetes: a statement of the American Diabetes Association. Diabetes Care 2005;28(1):186–212.
28. Twyman S, Rowe D, Mansell P, et al. Longitudinal study of urinary albumin excretion in young diabetic patients – Wessex Diabetic Nephropathy Project. Diabet Med 2001;18:402–8.
29. Lutale JJ, Thordarson H, Avvas ZG, et al. Microalbuminuria among type 1 and type 2 diabetic patients in Dar Es Salaam, Tanzania. BMC Nephrol 2007;15(8):2. Available at: http://www.ncbi.nlm.nih.gov/pubmed/17224056?ordinalpos=8& itool=EntrezSystem2. Accessed September 12, 2008.
30. Palmer Alves T, Lewis J. Racial differences in chronic kidney disease (CKD) and end-stage renal disease (ESRD) in the United States: a social and economic dilemma. Clin Nephrol 2010;74(Suppl 1):S72–7.
31. Moayeri H, Dalili H. Prevalence of microalbuminuria in children and adolescents with diabetes mellitus type 1. Acta Med Iran 2006;44(2):105–10.
32. Ferrari P. Prescribing angiotensin-converting enzyme inhibitors and angiotensin receptor blockers in chronic kidney disease. Nephrology (Carlton) 2007;12:81–9.

Strategies from Bedside Nurse Perspectives in Conducting Evidence-based Practice Projects to Improve Care

Susan T. Shaffer, RN[a,*], Colleen D. Zarnowsky, BSN, RN[a],
Renee C. Green, BSN, RN[a], Mei-Lin Chen Lim, BSN, RN, CCRC[a],
Brenda M. Holtzer, PhD, RN, PCNS-BC[b], Elizabeth A. Ely, PhD, RN[a]

KEYWORDS

- Evidence-based practice • Research Utilization • Practice change
- Bedside Nurses and staff nurses • Pain Management • Magnet
- Quality Improvement

KEY POINTS

- The evidence-based practice (EBP) process may take longer than anticipated.
- Identify and involve staff nurses who have an interest in the project. The group should ideally include 5 to 8 nurses, depending on the scope of the project.
- Involve clinical and research experts to help identify the scope of the project, assist with the process, and establish a realistic timeline to understand the concept and to plan accordingly.
- Identify and follow an EBP model that all can easily understand and use.
- Set goals and a timeline. Be prepared to modify the timeline as needed.
- Communicate the plan not only to each member of the team but also to the nurse manager and all appropriate staff members responsible for project implementation.

Supporting bedside nurses to conduct evidence-based practice (EBP) projects at the point of care is desirable, especially in the climate of hospitals working to achieve Magnet Recognition.[1] Exploring barriers and facilitators encountered when bedside

Funding sources: No extramural funding or commercial support received for this project.
Conflict of interest: The authors disclose that there is no conflict of interest related to this project.
[a] Department of Nursing, The Children's Hospital of Philadelphia, 34th Street and Civic Center Boulevard, Philadelphia, PA 19104, USA; [b] Penn State Abington, 1600 Woodland Road, Abington, PA 19001-3990, USA
* Corresponding author.
E-mail address: shaffers@email.chop.edu

http://dx.doi.org/10.1016/j.cnur.2013.01.004
0029-6465/13/$ – see front matter
nursing.theclinics.com

nurses initiate and carry out an EBP project enhances nursing leadership's knowledge about the issues for promoting participation of nurses at the bedside.

BACKGROUND

The Magnet Recognition Program was developed to recognize organizations providing excellence in nursing practice.[1] The hallmark characteristics of Magnet designation include empowering nurses for autonomous practice and emphasizing critical inquiry, development of new knowledge to improve quality care, and the need to examine and improve outcomes. Involving nurses at all levels of practice to explore the evidence base for the nursing care they provide helps to strengthen knowledge, promote excellence, and ensure quality.[2]

Much has been published about the challenges of research use for busy staff nurses. Application of EBP by nurses at the point of care includes challenges such as lack of time, resources, and organizational support.[3–9] Carlson and Plonczynski[5] recently conducted an integrative review of 45 studies to determine the influence of the Barriers to Research Utilization Scale (BARRIERS scale) on nursing practice. The investigators concluded that identified barriers to research use have remained the same over the past 15 years. They added that the focus needs to shift to examining the relationship between perceived barriers and the uptake of EBP practice change.

Spenceley and colleagues[10] also conducted an integrated review examining the sources of information used by nurses to inform their practice. Nurses tended to rely on informal sources such as their peers for expert clinical advice, suggesting that any successful approach to integrating evidence into practice needs to be unit based. Integration of EBP may be more successful when engaging nurses at the point of care in identification of clinical problems and assisting them to evaluate and incorporate the best evidence into their practice.

Our institution, The Children's Hospital of Philadelphia (CHOP), is committed to supporting Magnet principles to strengthen nursing practice. The challenge of putting these principles into action is discussed in this article. The purpose is to provide insight into the process of identification of a clinical issue and creating change through a thorough review of evidence resulting in policy modification with implementation of the change into practice. Bedside nursing staff played an integral role in the process from start to finish.

EBP PROJECT: PAIN ASSESSMENT TOOL FOR CHILDREN WITH COGNITIVE IMPAIRMENT

The EBP project team was formed from a committee of CHOP nurses with an interest in improving pain management. The committee, Pain Resource Nurses (PRN), has representation from staff across all specialty practice, inpatient, and some outpatient settings. The PRN group derived from The Department of Nursing, Shared Governance council, Quality, Practice, and Patient Safety. There is strong evidence to support the development of a pain nurse expert or PRN model as a way to effectively improve pain management for hospitalized patients.[11,12]

As the PRN group prioritized methods to improve the quality of pediatric pain care, the lack of a pain assessment tool for children with cognitive impairment (CI) stood out. A core group of nurses consisting of bedside nurses, a clinical nurse specialist (CNS), a research nurse coordinator, and a nurse researcher formed the EBP project team to identify a comprehensive pain assessment tool for use with this population. The project team followed steps of the EBP process, a quality-improvement (QI) project, and implementation of the chosen pain assessment tool into policy and practice. The guiding principles of the Johns Hopkins Nursing EBP (JHNEBP) model of evidence and translation represented the steps followed by the project team.[6] Details on the review of the literature on 9 published pain assessment tools for children with CI and the QI project have been published.[13,14] See **Fig. 1** for a summary of the steps undertaken by this project team. The pain assessment tool for children with CI selected was the Revised Faces, Legs, Activity, Cry, and Consolability (rFLACC) scale.[15] The rFLACC includes behaviors based on evidence to represent pain for children with CI.[16] There is also a section that allows parents to add behaviors identified specifically for their child. The Faces, Legs, Activity, Cry, and Consolability (FLACC) scale does not include behaviors specific to CI. The EBP project, Pain Assessment Tool for Children with Cognitive Impairment, is used here to illustrate the experiences of bedside nurses that influenced a hospital-wide change for the improvement of nursing care for a vulnerable group of pediatric patients.

FACILITATING FACTORS

Juggling bedside care with other project responsibilities posed challenges personally and professionally.[7] The philosophy of the CHOP Department of Nursing promotes bedside nurses to conduct scholarly activities by providing resources for guidance

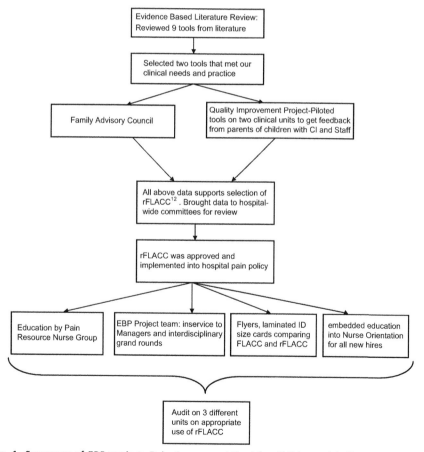

Fig. 1. Summary of EBP project: Pain Assessment Tool for Children with Cognitive Impairment. FLACC, Faces Legs Activity Cry and Consolability; rFLACC, revised FLACC.

and online educational modules to support knowledge gaps. Along with these resources, other facilitating factors need to be present to carry out a project from conception to after implementation. Facilitating factors that promoted the process and outcomes of this EBP project are reviewed in detail later.

Motivation to Provide Optimal Care

Interest in determining best practices for pain management for children with CI was a strong motivating factor. Children with CI are admitted to most inpatient units where their medical and surgical needs often include pain management. When caring for children with CI, providing optimal care for pain requires observation and close communication with the parent/guardian of the child. Bedside nurses from the PRN group acknowledged that a different approach to pain assessment for this population was needed to provide the best possible care. Using evidence-based best practice to provide optimal pain management for this vulnerable population of children was recognized as essential by project team members. Because providing pain management for this population poses challenges to nurses, the EBP project was an opportunity to have a positive impact on a known area for improvement. With guidance from clinical and research experts, it was determined to first review the literature and identify a valid, reliable pain assessment tool specifically developed for children with CI that included close collaboration with parents/guardians.

Professional Factors

Another motivating factor for involvement in the project was professional development. In addition to the coauthors' bedside nurse roles, they also serve leadership roles within their units. Participation in the EBP project provided hands-on experience to conduct a literature review, learn the EBP process, and to improve pain management for this group of patients. Professional development for project team members involved the desire to strengthen leadership skills by encouraging critical thinking through evidence review and synthesis to produce change in patient care. At the start, team members had limited experience with literature and evidence review and wanted to learn more about EBP and pain management for children with CI. The bedside nurses involved chose to spend time outside their work hours to complete certain project tasks such as writing of the manuscripts. The desire to be involved in a process that would produce a hospital-wide change and the ability to strengthen leadership skills were some of the strong motivating factors that supported nurses throughout the project.

Support and Guidance

Expert support and guidance was required to facilitate the bedside nurses' project involvement.[8] The project team's nurse researcher, nurse research coordinator, and CNS provided guidance on how to conduct the project, including establishing project timeline, education on knowledge gaps, and strategies necessary to implement a hospital-wide practice change. The nurse managers supported the project team's bedside nurses' involvement by providing coverage to attend project team meetings and allowing project time to complete literature review and coordinate the unit-based QI pilot. During the pilot, each unit developed its own methods to identify and complete the QI project tasks. Unit-specific staff nurses were enlisted to support tasks such as identifying appropriate patients to trial the published pain assessment tools within the units. Bedside nurse team members acted as unit-based change agents. They were crucial in facilitating their nursing colleagues' engagement and participation. Because the bedside nurses involved had no previous experience in a project of this magnitude, these supportive relationships were key to the success of the project. In summary, the strengths of involving staff nurses in EBP work included increasing knowledge of the staff nurses on EBP, promoting the professional growth of the nurses involved, and gaining commitment from the nursing staff.

BARRIERS AND STRATEGIES TO CONDUCTING EBP

Although there are many good reasons to work on a project that can positively affect caring for children in pain, there are barriers that can hinder the successful completion of the project. The following discussion examines some of those barriers and explains how the project team devised solutions to overcome them.

Time

The first barrier that the bedside nurses needed to overcome was a lack of time.[4,9] Patient care is a priority in health care institutions. The bedside nurses found it a challenge to have committed blocks of time away from patient care. A project timeline to plot meetings and deadlines was essential. Meeting with the subgroup meant additional time away from patient care. Working with each nurse manager, the bedside nurses needed to advocate for time to work on the project.[8]

Staff nurses at CHOP get time to work on nondirect patient care needs, called project time. However, the time may be limited or variable depending on patient care needs, census, acuity, vacations, staffing, and other preplanned classes and committee meetings. Many factors are considered when managers or schedulers determine vacation, class, or project time. There is a guideline of allowing only 10% of full-time equivalents off at 1 time. The scheduler considers the specific requests for project time and fills it in on shifts in which it can be accommodated. Staff nurses who are committee members or teach classes have prescheduled time. In order for the project team's bedside nurses to get approval for the project work time, each of them maintained communication with their respective nurse managers regarding the project's progress and the projected work needed to conduct the EBP process. Key to continued manager support was evidence of meeting established project deadlines. Balancing patient care, unit responsibilities, and the EBP project was difficult at times.

The employment status of being part time or full time posed advantages and disadvantages for the bedside nurses. The bedside nurses' schedules and shifts were variable, which presented some difficulties in scheduling project meeting times when all could be present. One of the advantages of being part time was schedule flexibility. Coming in on an unscheduled day or staying after the end of shift enabled the time to complete project tasks such as review of articles, coordination and monitoring of progress of the QI pilot, and auditing the postimplementation use of the tool. The disadvantages were not being there consistently to gather data or to follow up with staff. The full-time bedside nurses could be there to monitor adherence but did not have the flexibility to juggle individual schedules to come in for a meeting or stay after a scheduled shift to work on data collection. Many times the bedside nurses called in from home for a meeting either to review an article or evaluate project progress. Dedication and accountability to commit their own time were necessary to complete the review of literature, organize the QI pilot, synthesize the data, and evaluate the use of the tool.

Knowledge

Lack of knowledge about how to participate in an EBP project was another barrier that the bedside nurses encountered.[3] There were struggles with reading and analyzing the literature, and being able to conceptualize and verbalize evaluation of the information. However, CNS and nurse researchers assisted the bedside nurses with literature search, review, and evaluation. It would have been difficult to accomplish the project without their expertise, support, and guidance.

Nursing Staff Commitment to Practice Change and Policy Adherence

Gaining commitment from staff nurses was another barrier that the project team faced. Because staff nurses did not participate in the literature review, they did not have the knowledge base necessary to support the bedside nurses involved in the project. Once the policy was changed and implemented to include the rFLACC tool for use with children with CI, not all staff nurses embraced the change and there were differing opinions on how to use the new assessment tool. For example, staff had difficulty identifying patients who were appropriate for use of the rFLACC versus the FLACC scale, which they were familiar using. Immediate postimplementation audit showed less-than-optimal uptake on use of the tool. Nurses often resorted to previous methods of pain assessment. Ongoing education by project team members and the PRN group provided clarification and rationale for using the rFLACC. One-to-one consultation was often used as an effective communication strategy for practice change. Involving all staff nurses from the beginning and explaining the EBP process and the tasks involved would have helped support the implementation of the project, the final policy, and the chosen assessment tool.

The project team bedside nurses did not have the ability to monitor adherence throughout the institution. They relied on each other to monitor their own unit's practice. The 2 pilot units were more successful with implementation and policy adherence. They had trialed the assessment tools and therefore were comfortable using them. In order to address the overall problem of lack of adherence, bedside nurses enlisted the help of other members of the PRN group in promoting the new tool on their own units. The help of other members of the PRN group was useful in promoting the new tool on their own units. A hospital-wide designated group or representative who promotes and monitors compliance on practice changes would have been helpful from the start of the implementation. During the time of this project, the electronic medical record was being built. The implemented pain assessment tool, rFLACC, was added to the electronic medical record pain assessment documentation and was key to sustaining the use of this tool.

LESSONS LEARNED

The project team bedside nurses have several recommendations to increase satisfaction and success when working on an EBP project:

- Plan for constant open communication using a variety of mechanisms.
- Frequently review the timeline and progress toward completion with the nurse manager and renegotiate project time as needed.
- Regularly update the nurse manager on progress toward project outcomes.
- Involve staff nurses early in the process so they understand and support the project purpose.
- Explain the process in staff meeting forums, provide articles that were reviewed, and update staff nurses on the process.

Although this project took longer than initially anticipated, the project team bedside nurses gained knowledge of the EBP process and the involvement required for hospital-wide change. They showed leadership internally by presenting at interdisciplinary grand rounds and locally within the units. The team effort also led to various opportunities of presenting at national conferences such as the American Nurses

Credentialing Center National Magnet Conference, Society of Pediatric Nursing Conference, and the International Association for the Study of Pain. Different team members took part in the scholarly activities and all were involved in manuscript writing and authorship. Along with the benefits of project participation, the project team's bedside nurses continue to strive to find new ways to promote the assessment tool and to monitor its use.

DISCUSSION

Bedside nurses' involvement in embedding change into practice occurred because nurses at the point of care saw value in implementing a change to improve pain management for a vulnerable group of patients in their care. Nurses at the bedside are best able to identify clinically significant practice concerns.[17] Creating systems to support and assist nurses helps to overcome the challenges and allow nurses to carry EBP projects to completion.[18–20] The rewarding experience leads to empowerment, increase in nurse satisfaction, and retention of highly effective staff in this ever-changing health care arena.

As has been discussed in the literature, a major barrier to nurses adopting EBP change is lack of time because of the increased complexity of patient care demands.[3,5,21] Some of the successes noted with this project included support at the individual, unit, and organizational level. At the core was discovering new knowledge to apply interventions (rFLACC pain assessment tool) in practice (improving pain management of children with CI). Project time was negotiated individually with unit leaders, although personal time was also needed to complete work. Having a core group of nurses working together and assisting each other was crucial because differing demands at times meant one nurse might have to take on more of the workload. Resources both in terms of time and personnel were crucial to success. Expertise from the Center for Pediatric Nursing Research and a unit-based CNS provided structure, education, and side-by-side assistance to the group. In addition, they helped the bedside nurses with evidence synthesis, pilot design and execution, and data analysis and interpretation.[19,20]

This work occurred with nurses from several clinical nursing units. Unit culture and a climate of leadership support at the unit level for project time were keys to success.[22] The subsequent involvement of PRN nurses from across the institution with common goals to improve pain management for children with CI helped with engaging staff, auditing practice, and ultimately sustaining the change.

Organizational support came from all leadership levels. Because the organization has been Magnet designated since 2004, there is a strong commitment to Magnet principles from the Chief Nursing Officer, directors, and managers in the Department of Nursing. Professional development rewards for the individual nurses and project group also reflected on the organization through national dissemination of the work and publication.

In conclusion, the bedside nurses recommend the following to other bedside nurses when considering starting an EBP project aimed at practice improvement and change:

- Realize that the EBP process will take longer than anticipated.
- Identify and involve staff nurses who are invested in the project. The group should include 5 to 8 nurses, depending on the scope of the project.
- Involve clinical and research experts to help identify the scope of the project, assist with the process, and establish a realistic timeline to understand the concept and to plan accordingly.
- Identify an EBP model to follow that all can easily understand and use.

- Set goals and a timeline. Be prepared to modify the timeline as needed.
- Communicate the plan not only to each member of the team but also to the nurse manager and all appropriate staff members responsible for project implementation.
- Remember the following 3 key words: time, patience, and perseverance.

SUMMARY

A bottom-up approach with the necessary organizational support and expertise from all levels of leadership assisted bedside nurses to complete this EBP project. Interventions aimed at research use can be successful when mindful of commonly understood barriers to completion, with steps taken to resolve those barriers.

REFERENCES

1. American Nurses Credentialing Center (ANCC). The Magnet model components and sources of evidence. American Nurses Credentialing Center. Silver Spring (MD): Author; 2008.
2. Luzinski C. An innovative environment where empowered nurses flourish. J Nurs Adm 2012;42(1):3–4.
3. Breimaier HE, Halfens RJ, Lohrmann C. Nurses' wishes, knowledge, attitudes and perceived barriers on implementing research findings into practice among graduate nurses in Austria. J Clin Nurs 2011;20(11–12):1744–56.
4. Brown CE, Wickline MA, Ecoff L, et al. Nursing practice, knowledge, attitudes and perceived barriers to evidence-based practice at an academic medical center. J Adv Nurs 2009;65(2):371–81.
5. Carlson CL, Plonczynski DJ. Has the BARRIERS scale changed nursing practice? An integrative review. J Adv Nurs 2008;63(4):322–33.
6. Newhouse RP, Dearholt SL, Poe SS, et al. Johns Hopkins nursing evidence-based practice model and guidelines. Indianapolis (IN): Sigma Theta Tau International; 2007.
7. Higgins I, Parker V, Keatinge D, et al. Doing clinical research: the challenges and benefits. Contemp Nurse 2010;35(2):171–81.
8. Ploeg J, Davies B, Edwards N, et al. Factors influencing best-practice guideline implementation: lessons learned from administrators, nursing staff, and project leaders. Worldviews Evid Based Nurs 2007;4(4):210–9.
9. Solomons NM, Spross JA. Evidence-based practice barriers and facilitators from a continuous quality improvement perspective: an integrative review. J Nurs Manag 2011;19(1):109–20.
10. Spenceley SM, O'Leary KA, Chizawsky LL, et al. Sources of information used by nurses to inform practice: an integrative review. Int J Nurs Stud 2008;45(6):954–70.
11. McCleary L, Ellis JA, Rowley B. Evaluation of the pain resource nurse role: a resource for improving pediatric pain management. Pain Manag Nurs 2004;5(1):29–36.
12. Paice JA, Barnard C, Creamer J, et al. Creating organizational change through the pain resource nurse program. Jt Comm J Qual Patient Saf 2006;32(1):24–31.
13. Ely E, Chen-Lim ML, Zarnowsky C, et al. Finding the evidence to change practice for assessing pain in children who are cognitively impaired. J Pediatr Nurs 2012;27(4):402–10.

14. Chen-Lim M, Zarnowsky C, Green R, et al. Optimizing the assessment of pain in children who are cognitively impaired through the quality improvement process. J Pediatr Nurs 2012;27:750–9.
15. Voepel-Lewis T, Merkel S, Tait AR, et al. The reliability and validity of the Face, Legs, Activity, Cry, Consolability observational tool as a measure of pain in children with cognitive impairment. Anesth Analg 2002;95:1224–9. http://dx.doi.org/10.1097/00000539-200211000-00020.
16. Malviya S, Voepel-Lewis T, Burke C, et al. The revised FLACC observational pain tool: improved reliability and validity for pain assessment in children with cognitive impairment. Paediatr Anaesth 2006;16:258–65.
17. Boyington AR, Ferrall SM, Sylvanus T. Marketing evidence-based practice: what a CROC! Clin J Oncol Nurs 2010;14(5):653–5.
18. Doran DM, Sidani S. Outcomes-focused knowledge translation: a framework for knowledge translation and patient outcomes improvement. Worldviews Evid Based Nurs 2007;4(1):3–13.
19. Gerrish K, Nolan M, McDonnell A, et al. Factors influencing advanced practice nurses' ability to promote evidence-based practice among frontline nurses. Worldviews Evid Based Nurs 2012;9(1):30–9.
20. Ingersoll GL, Witzel PA, Berry C, et al. Meeting magnet research evidence-based practice expectations through hospital-based research centers. Nurs Econ 2010; 28(4):226–35.
21. Koehn ML, Lehman K. Nurses' perceptions of evidence-based nursing practice. J Adv Nurs 2008;62(2):209–15.
22. Rycroft-Malone J. Leadership and the use of evidence in practice. Worldviews Evid Based Nurs 2008;5(1):1–2.

Index

Note: Page numbers of article titles are in **boldface** type.

Moving?

Make sure your subscription moves with you!

To notify us of your new address, find your **Clinics Account Number** (located on your mailing label above your name), and contact customer service at:

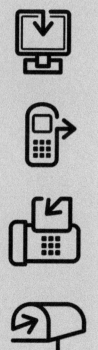

Email: journalscustomerservice-usa@elsevier.com

800-654-2452 (subscribers in the U.S. & Canada)
314-447-8871 (subscribers outside of the U.S. & Canada)

Fax number: 314-447-8029

Elsevier Health Sciences Division
Subscription Customer Service
3251 Riverport Lane
Maryland Heights, MO 63043

*To ensure uninterrupted delivery of your subscription, please notify us at least 4 weeks in advance of move.

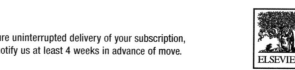

Printed and bound by CPI Group (UK) Ltd, Croydon, CR0 4YY

08/06/2025

01896873-0012